The
Pilates
Bible

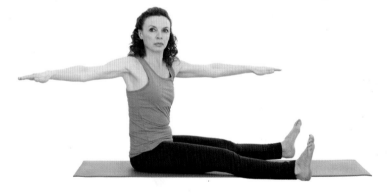

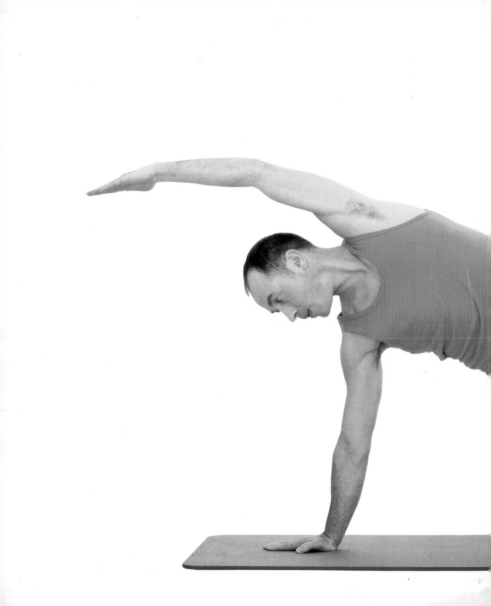

The
Pilates
Bible

Jo Ferris

The definitive guide to Pilates exercises

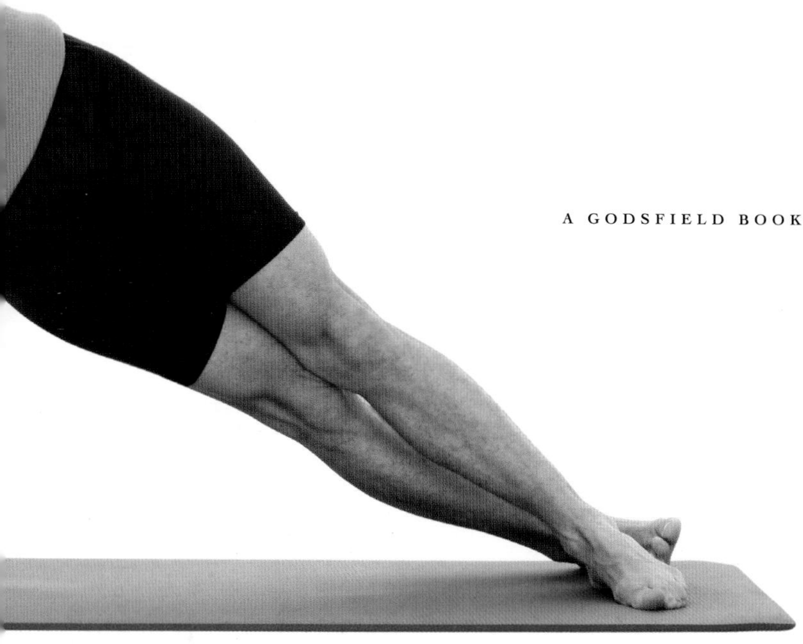

A GODSFIELD BOOK

First published in Great Britain in 2013 by Godsfield Press, a division of Octopus Publishing Group Ltd • www.octopusbooks.co.uk

ISBN 978-1-59120-317-9

10 9 8 7 6 5 4 3 2 1

Publisher Liz Dean
Consultant Editor Gerry Maguire Thompson
Art Director Yasia Williams-Leedham
Photography Ruth Jenkinson
Senior Editor Sybella Stephens
Models Benji Vize Harrington, Carly Best, Francis Christeller, Shahla Tarrant and Zoe Ayling

Contents

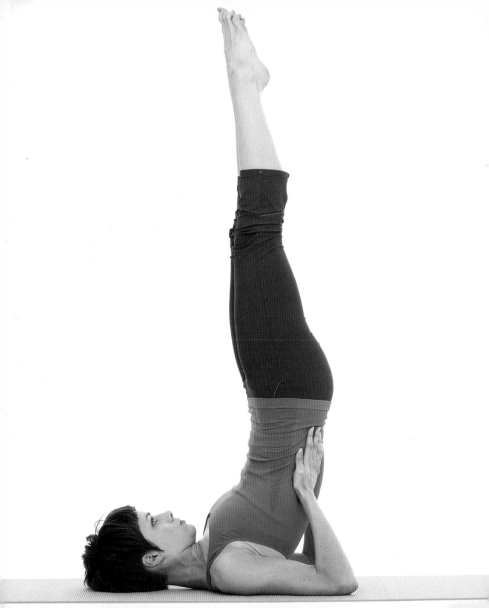

Introduction

This book aims to be a comprehensive adjunct to your journey in learning Pilates. Nothing can replace the watchful and skilled eye of a good instructor, and it is certainly worth the investment of learning with one. However, practice on your own is essential. This book will help guide you in your personal practice, and will consolidate what you learn in your sessions with an instructor. Combining individual practice with professional instruction offers a powerful combination: you will grow stronger and fitter more quickly, enabling you to reap the rewards in your everyday life.

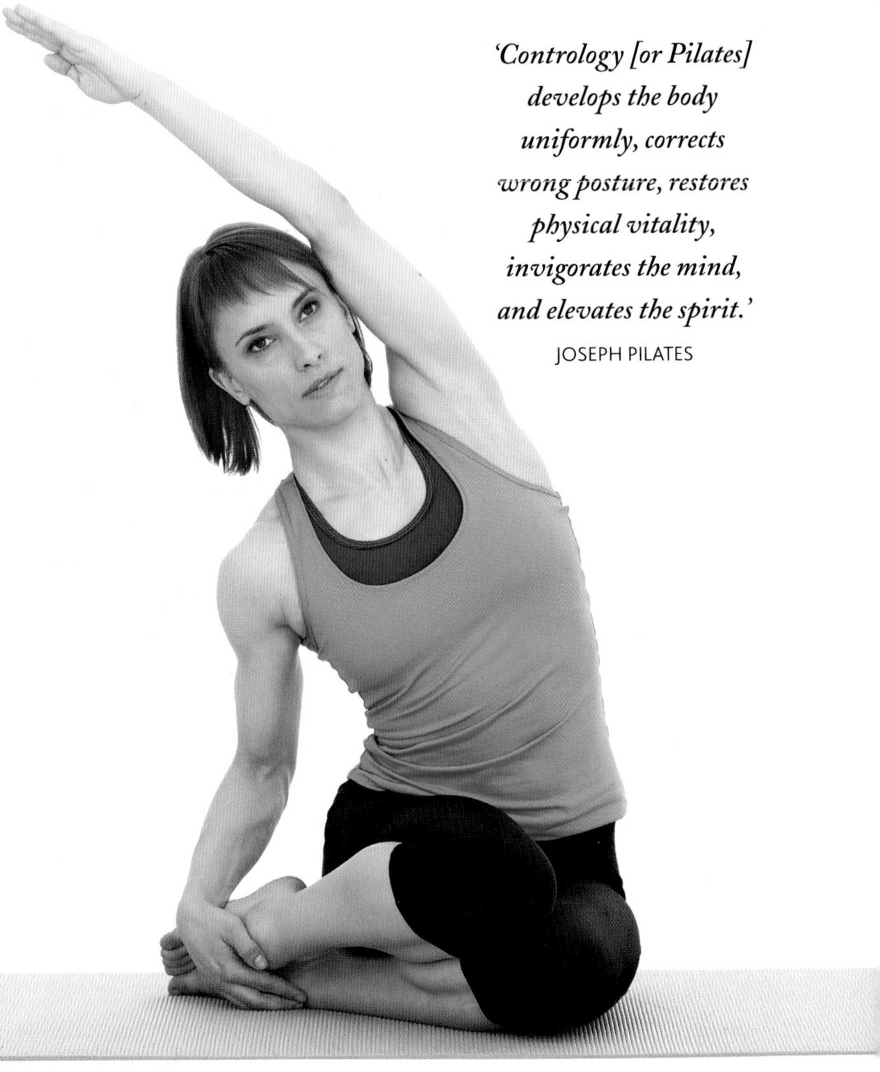

'Contrology [or Pilates]
develops the body
uniformly, corrects
wrong posture, restores
physical vitality,
invigorates the mind,
and elevates the spirit.'

JOSEPH PILATES

Why do Pilates?

What better reason do you need to start Pilates than the opposite statement? Joseph Pilates (1880–1967) designed his exercise system to work every muscle in the body, in order to improve the circulation of the blood to every fiber and tissue of the body, with all the benefits that improved circulation will bring.

Joseph Pilates taught the individual in front of him and, as each person has a different body, no one person was taught in exactly the same way as any other. The system is therefore highly adaptable, which enables it to be accessible to most people, regardless of their starting level of fitness. Someone recovering from injury and the elite athlete alike can use Pilates to enhance their body strength and fitness.

The connection of mind and body is one huge benefit brought about by the Pilates system. It is well recognized that exercise increases the release of endorphins (naturally occurring chemicals released by the brain during exercise that aid pain relief and produce feelings of well-being) and has the potential to lift your mood. Pilates has the added benefit of "gaining the mastery of your mind over the complete control of your body," intensifying the sense of well-being that is generated by this form of training.

In recent years Pilates has become increasingly popular, for it has the potential to strengthen your core stability and increase your flexibility and stamina. And, once you have mastered some of the movements, the structure of the Pilates system enables those benefits to be incorporated into your everyday life (see Chapter 9).

How to Use This Book

Pilates is not an exercise fad involving a series of separate and disconnected exercises; rather, it is a sophisticated movement system with a structure and purpose to everything it expounds. It is a very powerful system, with the potential—if you practice—to produce dramatic lifelong changes to your body. To achieve this, Pilates needs to be learned properly from the outset.

Joseph Pilates, the creator of this discipline, said: "In ten sessions you will feel a difference, in twenty you will see a difference and in thirty you will have a whole new body." In his book *Return to Life through Contrology* (as he called what we now know as Pilates) he expressed the belief that his system did not require membership of an expensive gym—his goal was to make the benefits of his system easily accessible to all. His "mat-work" was designed to be carried out in the home environment at only nominal cost to the individual, as long as the individual "conscientiously obeys" the instructions for every exercise.

THE IMPORTANCE OF STARTING AS A BEGINNER

The book—which will guide you in your personal practice, consolidating what you learn with an instructor—is designed to take you right from the very basics of Pilates, with preliminary exercises called the Fundamentals, through to the advanced mat workout. It is important to view learning Pilates, as a process, and to resist the temptation to skip straight to the dynamic challenging exercises in the Advanced Program. If you are already fit and strong, you may think it is okay to do this, but this is not so.

Having had experience of teaching Pilates over many years, I have taught people right across the spectrum—from those

The Beginner's Program will teach you the foundations for the more challenging parts of Pilates.

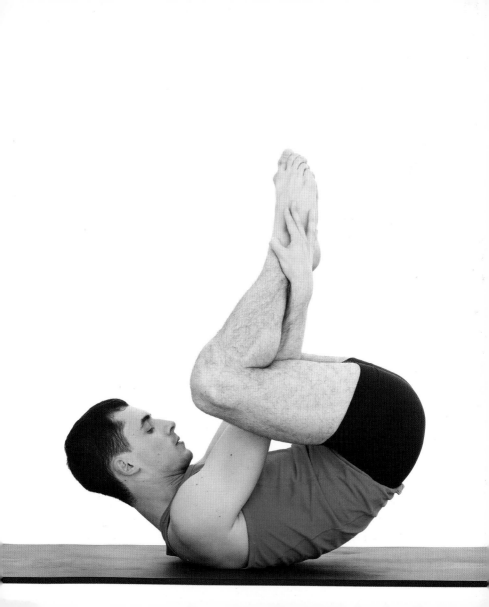

with injuries to the very fit. Being fit enough to run half-marathons does not mean that a student will have good core stability: a muscle-bound young man with well-defined abdominals will not necessarily have the core control to perform some of the more challenging Pilates exercises safely. Some athletic individuals who have focused solely on one sport may have difficulties with flexibility and limitations in their range of movement, which may prevent them performing some Pilates exercises unless they use some of the modifications that are provided in this book. Therefore *everybody*—regardless of their individual fitness level—needs to start at the very beginning.

Even the very fit need to learn Pilates from the beginning.

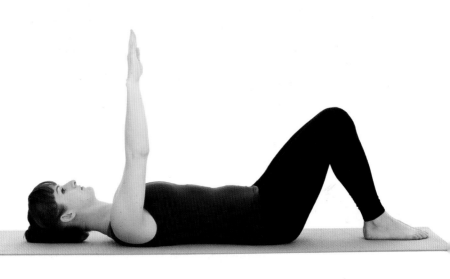

STAGES OF LEARNING

THE FUNDAMENTALS (see pages 58–83) will teach you how
to align yourself on the mat and how to "scoop" your abdominal muscles. *Do this section first*—do not progress until you
have these preliminary Pilates exercises programd into your
body.

THE BEGINNER'S PROGRAM (see pages 84–127) is a very
basic mat workout and gives you an opportunity to develop
into some simple movements what you have already programd into your body from the Fundamentals section. You
can thus begin to train the stamina of your core muscles,
combined with control and some flexibility.

Before you move on from the Beginner's Program you need
to be sure that you are ready to progress to the Intermediate
Program. You need to be able to perform any exercise safely
and effectively before challenging yourself further. Progression signs are indicators that you are strong
enough to move from one level to the next—
here are a few of those progression signs:

*Learning the
Fundamentals will
program essential
components of
movement into
your body.*

- The exercises should be pain-free! However, don't mistake the sense of effort and a sensation of gentle stretching for pain.
- You should be able to maintain your "scoop" (see page 28) and all your other connections throughout the move.
- You should be able to achieve and maintain the *Precision points* listed for each exercise.
- You should be able to perform the exercise without any of the *Common errors*.
- You should be consistent in achieving all of the above.

Progress by adding just one new move each time you practice a session, and build your proficiency with the new exercise before adding more.

Learning to lift your head correctly will help you engage your abdominals.

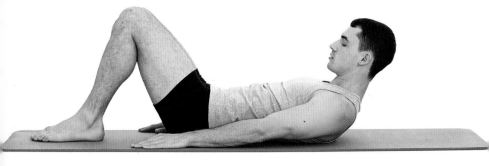

THE INTERMEDIATE PROGRAM (see pages 128–211) challenges your flexibility to a greater extent using your powerhouse (see page 28), and with connections worked through bigger movements and in different positions. You may need to work at this level for a while before moving onto the Advanced Program (see pages 212–349). Some students won't move on to the advanced section at all—the intermediate level will continue to challenge them sufficiently and provide goals to work toward. Don't make the transition to the advanced section in one leap; as before, introduce one new exercise at a time.

The intermediate program will begin to challenge your core control more deeply.

THE ADVANCED PROGRAM shows Pilates as it was intended to be: dynamic, strong and challenging. If performed in a controlled way, with proper execution, it is a safe form of exercise. If completed sloppily—without having learned Pilates properly, or by missing out the beginner's stages—there is the potential for injury, as with any demanding form of exercise. Being able to do 20 sit-ups and 30 press-ups does *not* mean that you are ready for the Advanced Program. Building the stamina required to complete the Abdominal Five and Push-Up series, with their limited number of repetitions, while scooped, and with all the parts of the body aligned, is a far greater challenge!

The advanced program takes your workout to the next level.

BACK AND NECK PROBLEMS

Pilates has gained a reputation for the rehabilitation of individuals who experience back and neck problems. The reasoning behind this link is sound, due to Pilates' ability to train the core muscles that help support the spine—a strong center gives a strong foundation for a strong, injury-free body.

The Beginner's Program is designed to work at a level that is suitable for most people recovering from injury, and includes *Modifications* to enable you to adapt the exercises further, as required. However, it is important to have permission from the members of your healthcare team before starting to exercise. Consult the professional who is most appropriately involved in the care of your back or neck—for instance, your doctor, physical therapist, chiropractor or osteopath.

SUMMARY OF HOW TO USE THIS BOOK

1 Read Chapter 1, paying particular attention to the Pilates principles (see pages 24–27).
2 Read Chapter 2, with particular reference to how to practice safely (see page 54) and how to work when recovering from injury (see page 53). Chapter 9 makes reference to more specific conditions and requirements in certain circumstances.
3 Learn the Fundamentals sequence in Chapter 3.
4 Start with the Beginner's Program in Chapter 4.
5 Check that you are ready to progress before challenging yourself further, with Chapters 5 and 6.

Enjoy the process!

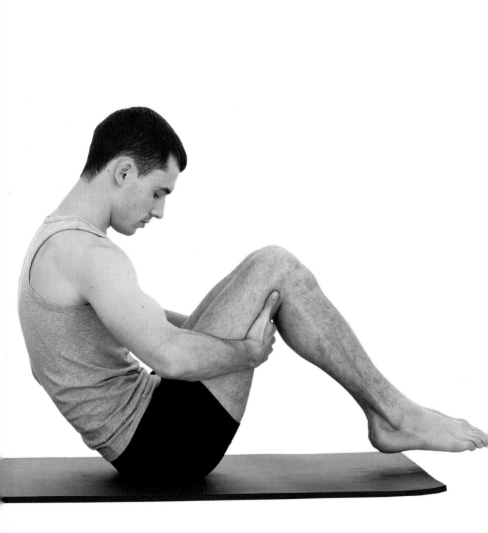

All About Pilates

This chapter will help you understand the origins of Pilates, how it works and how it can have an impact on your body. Reading about the principles and concepts behind Pilates will deepen your understanding of this exercise system and enhance the benefits that you will gain from practicing it.

History of Pilates

Pilates has its origins nearly a hundred years ago. Joseph Pilates was born in Germany in 1880, and his heritage was based on exercise and well-being—his father was a gymnast and his mother a naturopath. Joseph suffered a good deal of ill health as a child, including asthma and rickets, and used physical activity to build his strength; by the time he was 14 he was in sufficiently good shape to be hired to pose for anatomical charts.

He continued to study movement and physical fitness, with an interest in both Western and Eastern practices, and earned a living in self-defence training, boxing and as a circus performer. He was in the UK when the First World War broke out in 1914 and was imprisoned by the British government, along with many other German nationals, as a potential security risk. During his internment as a prisoner of war on the Isle of Man, Joseph continued to maintain his own fitness and developed training programs for the other inmates, to maintain their physical well-being—this was the beginning of the Pilates mat-work system. During the flu epidemic of 1918 the followers of his fitness technique remained free from flu, and Joseph expanded his technique to those inmates who were too unwell to leave their beds, adapting his program using springs and anything else which he could improvise with. These ideas were later incorporated into his development of Pilates equipment.

A GROWING REPUTATION

After the war Joseph returned to Germany, where he continued to develop his technique and built a reputation for getting good results with his exercise system, which was used by dancers and the German police force. In 1925 he left for the United States, after being asked to train the German army, which was inconsistent with his pacifist beliefs. He met his future wife, Clara, on the boat to New York and they set up their first studio in 1926, again teaching dancers as well as actors and athletes. Joseph's reputation continued to grow and his clients included high-profile artists from the dance world.

The Pilates system that we know today was originally called "Contrology," and the original form was the mat-work—Joseph Pilates' intention being that his system should be available to all, with little or no financial outlay. The equipment was developed for studio use and had the advantage of providing resistance, feedback and, at times, an added challenge.

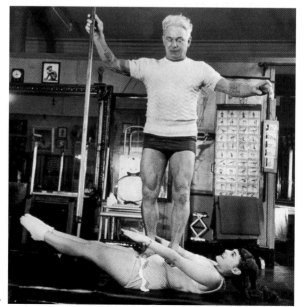

Joseph Pilates, 1951.

Classical Pilates

Joseph Pilates wrote two books about his exercise system: *Return to Life through Contrology* (1934) and *Your Health* (1945). *Return to Life Through Contrology* describes the principles behind his system, including the importance of breathing correctly, the interaction of mind and body, and the belief that health is holistic (that is, treating the whole person rather than specific illnesses and ailments) and requires a healthy mind and body. It also includes the 34 original mat exercises.

However, most of Pilates' work was passed on by several devoted followers whom Joseph taught and who have become known as the "Elders." Classical Pilates—as it was originally intended to be—has been preserved and passed down by these Elders, who have trained their own generation of teachers. The only changes to classical Pilates have come about when our understanding of movement, physiology or anatomy has progressed by means of scientific advances. Where the Pilates approach has descended outside the scope of the Elders, however, changes have been made to the system that may reflect the influences of the individuals or organizations involved.

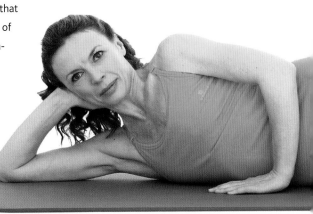

The side kick series of exercises challenges balance and stability.

VITAL PILATES COMPONENTS

A number of important components give classical Pilates its power, and provide the vital link between practicing Pilates and feeling the benefits in your everyday life. They are:

- The sequence and order of the exercises produce balance in the body.
- The idea of flowing movement, using transitions and linking one move to another, helps to improve stamina.
- The order of the exercises works *with* gravity: initially you lie down, as it is easier to work this way, changing posture so that you gradually end the session working upright, *against* gravity. This gently removes strain from the joints and gradually reloads them, teaching the body's core muscles in a progressive way.
- The system is very adaptable, accessible to most students (irrespective of their baseline fitness), yet creates demands and can challenge even the fittest body.
- Pilates is inspirational—always challenging students to be the very best they can be, by working as close to the ideal as possible.

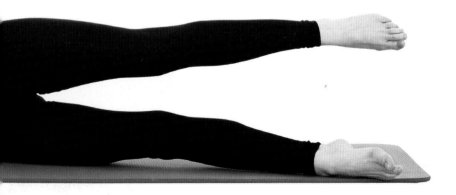

Pilates Principles

Joseph Pilates used six principles to inform and guide the student when working with his system. When applied, these principles give Pilates its power, taking the exercises from a set of movements to a holistic mind–body–spirit modality.

1: BREATHING

Breathing is vital for life, and for exercise. Working with ordinary people in everyday life has shown me how often faulty breathing patterns can become habitual, because of stress, anxiety, poor posture and lack of fitness.

For instance, it is common for people to breath-hold when they start an exercise with which they are not familiar. But holding your breath deprives the muscles of oxygen and can make exercising an uncomfortable—and unnecessarily effortful—process. It is most important to let the breath flow. Joseph Pilates was aware of the importance of one's breathing, stressing the significance of a full exhalation followed by a full inhalation, therefore maximizing oxygenation—the process by which oxygen is absorbed into the body.

The Pilates system is also cleverly designed so that breathing correctly helps the exercises to flow and fits with the shape of the exercise, removing any sense of jerkiness or discomfort. As a general principle, the out-breath always occurs at the point in the exercise when the body is flexed, rotated or bent (with the prompt of "wringing the lungs out" until there is no air left), while the in-breath generally accompanies the effort or occurs when the spine and body are lengthened. The way the breath works in Pilates reflects what we know about the diaphragm and the role that it plays in core stability. However, don't get too caught up in watching your breath—just remember to move and let your breathing flow!

> *'Breathing is the first act of life, and the last."*
> JOSEPH PILATES

2: CENTRING

In Pilates the term "core stability" was not originally used by Joseph Pilates, but he understood that a strong core in the center leads to a strong body; the term he used for the core was the "powerhouse." All movements are powered from this powerhouse, and this is a term that we shall use a lot throughout this book.

In Pilates an awareness of our centerline is also used to keep our movements correct and controlled. Everybody has an inherent awareness of where the centerline of their body is, and this helps to create an internal framework for where the body is in space. Working toward and from your centerline in your Pilates workout will enable you to find the correct connections in your body.

'Contrology is designed to give you suppleness, natural grace, and skill that will be unmistakably reflected in the way you walk, in the way you play, and in the way you work."
JOSEPH PILATES

The idea of a "center" is not just a physical concept. If you are "centerd" mentally while you move, you become more focused and more aware of what is happening within your body. With more focus, you will move with greater accuracy; this will remind your nervous system what it feels like to move naturally, and will enable the nervous system to generate more desirable movement patterns. To be mentally centerd during your Pilates session will raise the exercise from a physical workout to the level of complete coordination of mind, body and spirit.

3: CONTROL

Originally Joseph Pilates called his system Contrology. It is important to move with control rather than let movements be uncontrolled or ballistic—using momentum and with flailing limbs. To move out of alignment is to invite injury within the body. Alignment has been proven by recent research studies to optimize activity in the correct muscles: those that are needed in order to have a strong center—the muscles that make up the body's core.

Control is needed in order to learn the basics as well as more adventurous movements. The Fundamentals section of this book (see pages 58–83) teaches you how to gain stability while carrying out small movements of the limbs.

'Contrology begins with mind control over muscles."

JOSEPH PILATES

4: CONCENTRATION

Concentrating fully will help you become centerd and move with greater control. Focus on achieving the best you can during your Pilates session—don't let your mind wander into making a mental shopping list or ruminating on the day's events. Leave extraneous thoughts at the door as you enter the room and bring your attention to your body: how it feels, and how you can move to the best of your ability. Learning from what we understand about the body and how it controls movement, we know that the sensations we feel while moving are pivotal in learning new movements, so don't let distractions cloud or dilute those sensations.

'Concentrate on the correct movements each time you exercise, lest you do them improperly."

JOSEPH PILATES

5: PRECISION

In Pilates there are no careless or uncontrolled movements. Using concentration and centering, don't just complete the exercise—complete it to your very best, and move with precision. Even for those who are most proficient at Pilates, the journey is never finished. There is always a greater challenge to be experienced, always more to learn. One way to keep the sense of challenge is to work with precision: it increases the intensity of your workout. You can always improve on the way in which you complete an exercise. It should never feel easy!

'You must always faithfully and without deviation follow the instructions accompanying the exercises and always keep your mind wholly concentrated on the purpose of the exercises as you perform them."
JOSEPH PILATES

6: FLOWING MOVEMENT

Pilates reflects the way we move naturally in everyday life. There are no static holds, and the Pilates system is dynamic and creates flowing movement, which is the way the nervous system aims to control our body's movement. As Pilates students, the aim is to move effortlessly, with grace and without harsh, jerky movements. Each exercise should flow, and each exercise should flow to the next exercise using the *Transitions* provided between the exercises. The Transitions are just as important as the exercises themselves; they encourage you to keep your powerhouse engaged throughout the entirety of a workout. When you are able to work with flow and connect one exercise to another, then you will start to feel the benefits in your everyday life.

Key Concepts in Pilates

**There are a number of key Pilates concepts with which it is important to
become familiar before starting to exercise. So read through the following top-
ics and try and get a feel for these concepts.**

POWERHOUSE

All movements in Pilates initiate from the powerhouse. It is your core—a band
around your middle that pertains to your deep abdominal and back muscles,
pelvic floor and diaphragm, supported by the gluteal muscles of your hips and
your pelvis. The powerhouse stabilizes your torso and "powers" every move.

SCOOPING

Scooping is the action of pulling the abdominal muscles inward and upward.
It forms a key part of activating the powerhouse, and aims to help stabilize
the spine and decompress it during movement, and is an aid to good posture.
Scooping is important to avoid "bearing down" and letting the abdominals bulge.

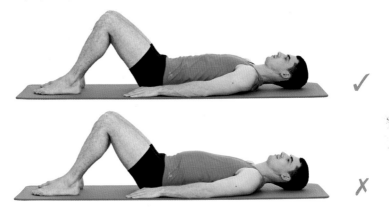

NEUTRAL SPINE/PELVIS

The position of the spine and pelvis is very important, particularly for core stability and engaging the deepest abdominal and back muscles. However, it is vital not to be distracted into making the position of the spine and pelvis the goal of these exercises. The spine is built for articulation as well as strength, and the pelvis needs to be free to move in relation to the spine and legs, to allow us to move flexibly. The key points when learning Pilates are to:

- Let the spine softly imprint itself on the mat: avoid letting it arch off the mat or bear down with bulging abdominals, forcing the back into the mat.
- Avoid tilting the pelvis so it is curled up and your tail bone is off the mat.
- Stabilize, both by scooping your abdominals and by having an active powerhouse.
- Imagine lengthening your spine from your tailbone to the crown of your head.

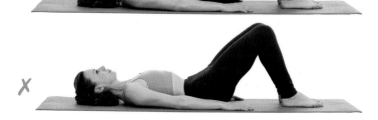

C-CURVE

In the instructions for the exercises throughout this book you will be directed to use your C-curve. This term is descriptive of the position that the spine adopts during certain exercises. To create it in your own body, pull your abdominal muscles deeply into your spine. The C-curve features in many different moves throughout the mat-work—for instance, in the set-up for exercises such as Rolling Like a Ball on page 98 and during a movement such as Spine Stretch Forward on page 108.

*Your abdominals
lift your spine to
create a C-curve.*

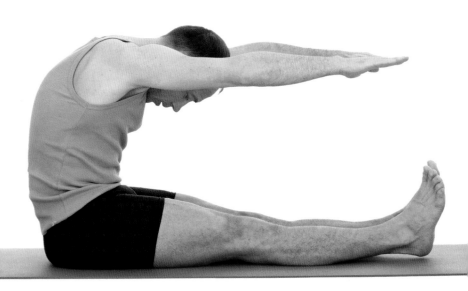

SPINAL ARTICULATION

The spine is built to articulate: for each vertebra to move relative to the next one. Pilates teaches flowing movements, which require a degree of mobility and flexibility; the spine needs to curl and uncurl during a series of movements in order to achieve the goal of the exercise safely. However, the spine may not be articulating freely, either due to areas of stiffness in the spine or due to weakness in the muscles that help control the movement of the spine. As Pilates is designed to improve mobility, control and strength, if you are centerd during your workout and are mindful of your body, then you will be able to improve the ability of your spine to roll up and down freely.

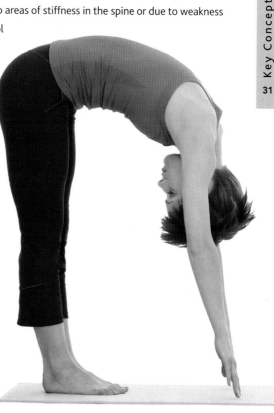

A healthy spine should be able to articulate freely.

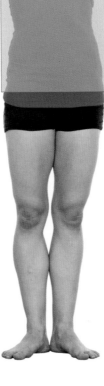

BOX

The concept of a box shape—from shoulder to shoulder and hip to hip—will increase your awareness of your alignment. Use this box as a tool to check on and correct your alignment.

Use the awareness of your box to move cleanly.

FRAME

The idea of a frame helps control your movement: your limbs should move safely within the frame of your body or the mat. The frame of your body is determined by the box of your body—the limbs should stay within the periphery of your vision; there should be no wild or uncontrolled movements of them.

LENGTH AND OPPOSITION

Pilates has become popular partly because the aesthetic results may include long, lean muscles, which create a pleasing shape and silhouette, as opposed to bulging muscles, which shorten the visual appearance of the limbs and trunk. The Pilates system achieves this in several ways. One of the most important is by teaching you to lengthen away from a stable center—that is, a strong powerhouse keeping the torso stable, enabling a limb to reach away in a lengthened position. The effect is to train muscles in their lengthened state as opposed to a shortened range, as in some other exercise methods such as bodybuilding.

CONNECTIONS

The descriptions in the exercises frequently refer to your "connections." Not only should your powerhouse be active, but if your other connections are working, they will help you become stronger and move with greater control. These other connections are:

- Rib and scapula (or shoulder blade) connection: the ribs are pulled in, flush with your front, and your shoulder blades are sitting in contact with the ribcage.
- Heel-to-seat connection: a sensation of your legs "zipping up" together, from your heel to your seat.
- Inner-thigh connection.

PILATES STANCE

The Pilates stance looks very much like a turning-out of the feet. However, as with everything in Pilates, it comes from the center and not from the periphery. The position is initiated with the backside and backs of the inner thigh muscles being active, creating a "wrap" of the upper legs and backside, which in turn helps support the powerhouse. The position of the legs naturally falls into place as a result of this; do not be tempted to think that you should stand in "first position" like a ballet dancer.

Pilates stance is also used in other positions, such as when the legs are in the air. In these positions don't point your toes— keep the points of your feet soft.

VISUALIZATION

Using imagery can be a very powerful aid in conveying the correct manner in which to move when learning an exercise. It can help connect the mind to the body and assist you in understanding the goal of an exercise, as well as increasing both performance and success. Using the *Visualizations* provided in the exercise descriptions will make your practice all the more effective.

CHIN TO CHEST

In many exercises that are performed lying on the mat on your back, your head is held up, with your eyes fixed on your navel. This helps to engage the powerhouse and

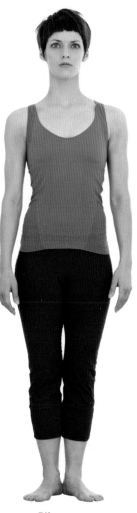

Pilates stance

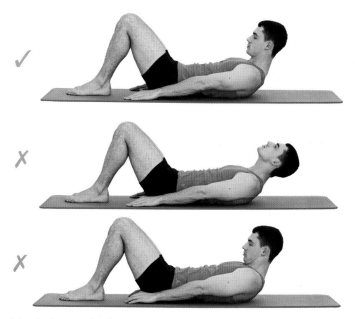

abdominals correctly. If your head is at the wrong angle, then your neck will feel strained and this will prevent your abdominals engaging properly. To lift your head, use your powerhouse and slide the front of your ribs into your waist; your eyes should look at your navel, and the front of your throat should stay soft and open, with just a small gap between the chin and the chest.

EFFORT WITH EASE

Our nervous system controls the way we move, always following a basic principle—it creates the most efficient movement possible, so that there is economy in the way we move, creating a smooth, seamless movement. During your Pilates workout your movements should be smooth, and should avoid clenching, bracing and strain. This is what we mean by the term "effort with ease." If you work at the exercise level that is correct for you, then your body will feel effort and challenge, but will still move freely.

How Pilates Works

CORE STABILITY

The Pilates system trains core stability. Very broadly, we can look at the body as having an "inner core" and an "outer core"; the inner core provides the spine and pelvis with stability, while the outer core helps in supporting the inner core, and moves the trunk. The Pilates system is constructed in such a way that, by practicing it, both your inner and outer cores will naturally be trained correctly.

INNER CORE

The inner core consists of the deep muscles that attach directly to every bone in the lumbar spine and deep into the pelvis. The inner-core muscles are:

- The deepest abdominal muscle, the transverse abdominis
- The very deepest back muscle, the multifidus
- The pelvic-floor muscles
- The diaphragm.

These muscles should maintain a background level of activity throughout the waking day, rather than isolated strong contractions and relaxations, in order to support the lumbar spine and the sacroiliac joints (where the spine joins the pelvis).

By being constantly active, these deep muscles provide stability and become slightly more active in anticipation of doing even the slightest movement, such as shifting position or lifting your hand to touch your face. This is necessary because the structure of the bones and ligaments in the spine does not provide sufficient stability on its own to withstand even the smallest increases of load on the spine; the spine is therefore dependent on the activity of these muscles to prevent instability or injury.

THE FOUR ABDOMINAL MUSCLES OF THE TRUNK

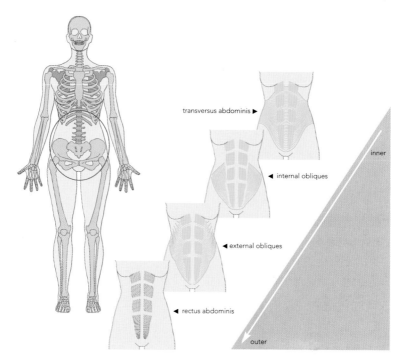

transversus abdominis ▶

inner

◀ internal obliques

◀ external obliques

◀ rectus abdominis

outer

The inner-core muscles work differently from the bigger, more visible muscles—they need to work at low levels of activity for prolonged periods of time, so they require high levels of stamina and must become more active before other muscles move the body, so they need to be trained differently. If you learn Pilates properly from the outset, with good instruction, then you will naturally learn to use your inner core.

THE REAR MUSCLES OF THE TRUNK SHOWING SOME OF THE MUSCLES THAT MAKE UP THE OUTER CORE

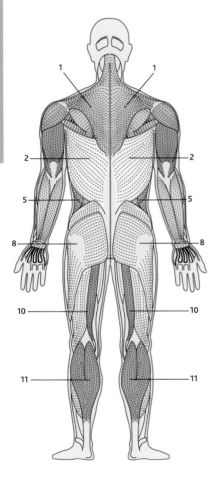

1 Trapezius—runs down the back of the neck and along the shoulders.

2 Latissimus dorsi—runs from the lower chest to the lumbar region. It draws the arm backward, pulls the shoulder down and back and the body upward.

3 Erector spinae (not shown)—this important muscle is at the back of the neck, chest and abdomen. It extends the spine and holds the body upright. When it acts on one side only it bends the spine to that side.

4 Transversus abdominis (not shown)—a deep internal muscle that runs across the abdomen. It holds the internal organs in place.

5 External oblique—side muscle of the abdomen. It compresses the abdomen and is used when moving the torso in any direction.

6 Rectus abdominis (not shown)—runs vertically down the front of the abdomen, supporting the internal organs and drawing the front of the pelvis upward.

7 Adductor—this inner thigh muscle draws the leg inward.

8 Gluteus maximus—forms part of the buttocks. It is important for maintaining an upright posture and in walking, running and jumping.

9 Quadriceps—runs down the middle of the front of the thigh. It acts in opposition to the semitendinosus.

10 Semitendinosus—one of the hamstrings. It runs down the middle of the back of the thigh and is used to extend the thigh and flex the knee.

11 Gastrocnemius—forming the greater part of the calf, this muscle runs down the back of the lower leg and is used in walking and running.

OUTER CORE

The outer core consists of the other abdominal muscles and back muscles, which are layered on top of the inner core. The oblique abdominal muscles are very much involved in supporting the inner core. Other large muscles of the trunk also form part of the outer core and help connect the pelvic and shoulder girdles to the trunk.

The muscles of the outer core help provide stability, but they cannot provide deep stability for the spine, as they are not attached to individual vertebrae. However, they do not only work in a stabilizing manner—they also move the body, so they need to be trained in such a way that they can stabilize and be strong enough to provide these big movements.

If your inner core becomes weak or is unable to function properly, then the big muscles on the surface of the body and trunk will become more dominant, to compensate. As we have just learned, these bigger muscles are unable to provide true stability to the spine and pelvis because they don't have deep attachments to the individual vertebrae; so if your inner core does not function properly, your body becomes vulnerable to pain and injury. In other words, a strong, well-functioning inner core enables stronger and more controlled movements of the limbs.

INTERACTION OF THE MUSCULOSKELETAL AND NERVOUS SYSTEMS

Good core stability is dependent upon more than muscles just being strong and active. To create stability the deep muscles have to be active before the body moves, and they also need to be active for prolonged periods of time, so the inner-core muscles need the nervous system to work efficiently to send out the right messages to the muscles. The nervous system ensures that the correct muscles are fired up, in the correct sequence and with the correct timing; it also uses information from all areas of the body—particularly from joints, muscles and ligaments—to send out the right messages to enable the body to move in a controlled way. If your core stability is not functioning properly, this may be due to the nervous system and muscular system not interacting correctly together. For your core stability to be robust, that interaction should be automatic and should not involve conscious thought. When you reach this point by practicing Pilates you will really begin to feel the benefits in your everyday life.

When the body moves spontaneously, muscles always work in pairs: to enable one muscle to contract, the opposing muscle needs to relax. Therefore to initiate a movement the nervous system never sends out messages to just one muscle—it also has to send out messages to stop another muscle working; and it sends messages to the inner-core muscles to stabilize the spine, before the stability of the spine is challenged. So the body never uses one muscle on its own, but works in patterns, in whole sequences of activating and deactivating muscles, to enable you to move. The nervous system controls this complex sequence.

Pilates not only trains movement, but also trains the nervous system to generate controlled, natural and desirable movement—true interaction between the nervous and musculoskeletal systems.

Benefits of Pilates

'The acquirement and enjoyment of physical well-being, mental calm and spiritual peace are priceless to their possessors, if there be any so fortunate living among us today." JOSEPH PILATES

MIND–BODY–SPIRIT CONNECTION

It is accepted that exercise has a positive effect on mood and our sense of well-being. Pilates cultivates "mindfulness"—being present in the here and now, to the exclusion of other distractions. By using the Pilates principles of concentration, centering, breathing, precision, flowing movement and control during your practice, you will begin to be able to shut out the outside world and any extraneous thoughts, and bring your focus to your body. This focus increases your body awareness, and a gentle balance between mind and body. Western medicine is beginning to appreciate the interaction between mind and body (and spirit)—each of which deeply affects the other. A healthily functioning physical state and exercise can have a great impact on our mental health, and equally our mental health can have a significant effect on our physical state.

COORDINATION

By practicing Pilates you will develop body awareness; and as your appreciation of where your body and limbs are in space improves, so the accuracy of the feedback to your nervous system will improve, leading to greater control of your movement.

Once you have learned the basics, you will find that the moves in Pilates have a rhythm and a dynamic that involve varying tempos. With practice, you will move in the "groove" of the exercise, and will enjoy the sensation of exercising with the sense of flow that comes with coordinated movement.

FLEXIBILITY

Pilates develops "stretch with strength." The flexibility gained in Pilates is achieved through a dynamic stretch, supported by what we know from science about movement control. Maximum contraction of a muscle or group of muscles is accompanied by maximum relaxation of the opposing muscle groups. An example of this is demonstrated in the Single Leg Kicks (see page 262), which provide an effective lengthening of the quadriceps muscles and hip flexors—by lying on your front, the hip joint is stabilized, and the muscles are already in a lengthened position; then, during the move, you contract your hamstrings and gluteal muscles to bend the knee, causing the quadriceps and hip flexors to "switch off" further, so allowing the knee to bend. The Pilates system incorporates movements in all dimensions for the spine and all the major joints, to enable the body to be free to move fluidly, without being impeded by tightness and stiffness.

CORE CONTROL

Core control comprises core stability and core strength. It is so important to learn Pilates properly from the outset, as the emphasis is on re-educating core stability, which often has to be learned in a very conscious way; if you skip to more advanced work too early on, you will miss out on this crucial process. As you progress, the system brings in many moves to train your core strength, and to train your core stability to become automatic—the way core stability should naturally occur when it functions normally.

Push-ups train strength in the arms and shoulders.

MUSCLE STRENGTH

Pilates mat-work trains strength in the muscles, by working those muscles along their whole length—not just when they are in their shortened position. Muscles don't just work by contracting to make the muscle shorter (known as "concentric activity"), but also by "paying out"—that is, by lengthening, once contracted ("eccentric activity"). In addition muscles are also able to work in two other ways; they can contract without changing length (an isometric contraction), and can maintain a contraction while the tension in the muscle remains the same but the muscle changes length (an isotonic contraction). These are all important ways in which muscles work.

To train the muscles correctly, they need to be trained in terms of the *way* they work. If a muscle's main function is to work eccentrically, then it needs to be trained in that way. Pilates mat-work naturally trains muscle groups in all the different ways in which they need to work, by using self-resistance (moving your limbs strongly and resisting your own movement), gravity and resistance from body weight (working against your own body weight in an exercise to increase the amount you have to work or the load to the muscles, e.g., press-ups or pull-ups).

POSTURE

In the work that I do as a Pilates teacher and physical therapist I am always watching how people move and observing their posture. I then mentally create a hypothesis for the reason for poor posture, as a deviation from the "normal." It is a fascinating occupation! In the 21st-century world that we inhabit a recurring phenomenon that I have observed is a combination of poking-out chin, rounded shoulders and a slumped, de-energized demeanour. We no longer have to hunt for our food, or even have to do all of our domestic chores manually. The net effect is that a large proportion of adults in the Western world spend a considerable amount of time seated, with hips and knees bent, spine flexed and the head falling forward from the neck. We leave our beds, get in the car and travel to work to spend eight hours at a desk, then return home to spend the evening seated on a comfy sofa. There are 168 hours in a week: what proportion of them do you spend in a slumped or recumbent position?

Poor posture places strain not only on our muscles, joints, ligaments and bones, but also on our respiratory, digestive and circulatory systems—potentially leading to headaches, altered breathing patterns and a sluggish digestive system. Over time, our bodies adapt to this less-desirable posture, leading to a loss of flexibility and making it harder to correct faulty posture; mild, niggling complaints may then become chronic issues.

Pilates, as an exercise system, is really well placed to have a positive impact on postural problems: it brings together work on all dimensions of the muscular and ligamentous systems, rather than training one body area, leading to overdevelopment and tightness. After a particular area of the body has been challenged or worked, it will often be stretched out in the next movement. A good example of this is the Teaser series (see page 196), which works the abdominals really hard; this is followed by Swimming (see page 200), where you lie on your front as you lengthen

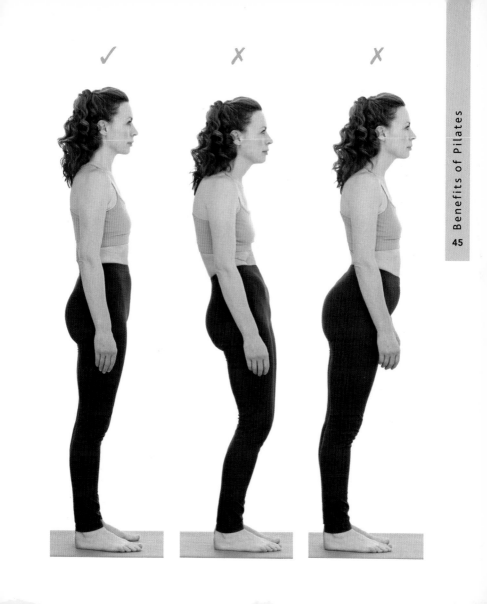

your abdominals. Pilates also tackles the areas of the body that often become tight due to altered posture; Double Leg Kicks, for instance (see page 264), opens up the fronts of the shoulders and chest—both of which are tight in a typical "poking-out-chin" posture.

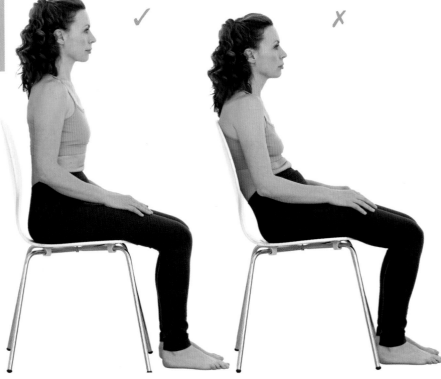

One often overlooked impact of poor posture is in the way individuals present themselves—stooped shoulders and a posture that conveys low levels of energy, for example, can give the impression of someone who is uninterested, even low in mood. Try it yourself: look in the mirror while standing with a poor, slumped posture and take note of your facial expression; consider the message you may be sending out to others. Now correct your posture or, better still, practice your Pilates routine; look back in the mirror again and see the difference: the person before you will appear more energized, your facial expression will have lifted and your whole demeanour will have "lightened"!

Poor posture will load your spine in a potentially damaging way.

Starting Pilates

Follow the guidance on starting Pilates given in this chapter, to get your journey off to the best start.

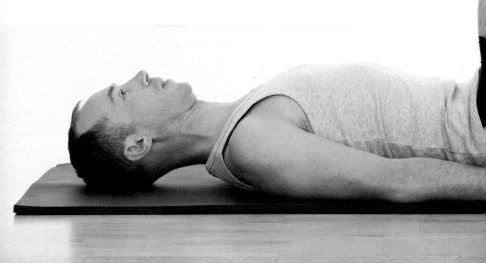

'*Study carefully.*
Do not sacrifice knowledge to
speed, in building your solid
exercise regime on the foundation
of Pilates. Follow instructions
exactly as indicated ... There is
a reason! Pilates is not a system
of haphazard exercises designed
only to produce bulging muscles.'

JOSEPH PILATES

Getting Started

You need very little in order to start Pilates: some space, a mat and, most importantly, the will, desire and motivation! If you have health issues, ensure that you have cleared yourself to exercise, by consulting your healthcare professional. If you are fit and well, then you are ready to begin.

In the Introduction (see pages 6–17) there was guidance on how to use this book. To recap, start with the Fundamentals section (see pages 58–83), which will teach you how to find your scoop and engage your powerhouse. It is absolutely *essential* that you have these basic skills, to enable you to practice Pilates safely and effectively. The Beginner's Program (see pages 84–127) is another important step in your learning process. If you are fit and already participate in other challenging forms of exercise, you might feel that this program will not work you hard enough; but, if done properly, the Beginner's Program will provide you with a challenge, and you will feel the work in your body. Do not skip these stages!

Pilates is a system with a structure, and there is good reason for the order of the exercises. One exercise will prepare your body for the following one; if it is omitted, then your body may not be warmed up or properly prepared for the subsequent exercise. The order of the exercises is also designed to cultivate muscle balance within the body, so if you choose to "cherry-pick" your own selection of exercises, your body may be denied one of the great therapeutic benefits of the Pilates system. So, in brief:

- Learn the Fundamentals.
- Don't be tempted to omit learning the Beginner's Program and race into the Intermediate or Advanced Programs.
- Stick to the order of the exercises within each level.

- Add in one exercise at a time as you progress, and slot it into the correct place; refer to Chapter 8, which gives you the complete mat workout.
- Use *Modifications* suitable for your level and your condition.
- Look for signs of your readiness to progress, as indicated in the exercise descriptions.
- Use the *Transitions* that are provided, to move between the exercises.
- Be mindful of your own body and how it feels.

The beginner's exercise Roll Down will teach you to articulate your spine by using your powerhouse.

WORKING TO YOUR THRESHOLD

We all have a limit to which we can exercise, regardless of our level of fitness. To improve our fitness we need to work at this threshold, which is the point at which we can just complete an exercise safely, while still maintaining the *Precision points* described in the text. The areas of fitness that are challenged at this threshold may include flexibility, stamina, strength, coordination, or a combination of these. Even the very fittest athlete has a threshold level to work at. Find your threshold level and work at that level. To push through that point will invite injury; to work below that level will limit your potential to benefit from your Pilates workout. This will become clearer when you embark on the exercises.

Whether a beginner or advanced, always work to your own level of fitness.

RECOVERING FROM INJURY

Pilates can be used in the rehabilitation phase after an injury, if it is done with awareness of safety, and if appropriate *Modifications* are adopted—these are described for the respective exercises. In the acute phase of an injury the correct management is to seek medical help, rest and follow the advice of your healthcare professional. Pilates is ideal for use as a tool for rehabilitation in the recovery phase, and for maintaining fitness if you are unable to participate in your regular sport or other physical activities. It is a low-impact exercise regime, and for the most part it removes the effect of gravity, thus reducing strain on the joints.

Rehabilitation is essential after an injury, to prevent a recurrence and any further lack of function. Pilates should be carried out under the supervision or guidance of a qualified practitioner; be advised by them concerning the right time to use Pilates for you. However, individuals also need to take responsibility for their own well-being, and rehabilitation activity need not necessarily be carried out in the presence of your healthcare practitioner—so follow their advice, but practice on your own too.

Pilates offers the opportunity to achieve several goals that frequently need to be achieved during rehabilitation:

- Core stability
- Flexibility
- Strength
- Stamina
- Proprioception: awareness of where the parts of your body are, and where the whole of your body is in space, helping to gain balance in the body and control of movement.

PRACTICING PILATES SAFELY

Pilates should never cause pain, but you should feel a sense of effort while you are practicing—if you don't, then you aren't working hard enough—and you will experience sensations of stretching. It is important to be able to distinguish between what is pain and what is simply effort or stretch. If anything feels sharp, burning or numb, it is wrong, so stop straight away!

There are, however, certain times when you should not practice Pilates. These are:

- When an injury is acute.
- If you are unwell with an infection or have a raised temperature.
- After a heavy meal or drinking alcohol. Aim to have eaten a small snack at least an hour or two before practicing, but avoid eating or drinking alcohol for the last hour before your Pilates session.
- When you are very fatigued. We all experience weariness from the pressures of everyday life, but this is not a reason not to practice Pilates; in fact it will energize you. However, there are times when fatigue is so great that it will put you at risk of injury if you exercise. Cultivating body awareness will guide you in this matter.

It is also very important to warm up. The Hundred exercise (see page 86) is designed to get your circulation going and to warm up your powerhouse, so don't leave it out. And use the Fundamentals (see pages 58–83) if you need a moment to clear your head and connect your mind to your body.

MODIFICATIONS

The instructions for each of the main exercises in this book list the goals of the exercise, how to perform it (in step-by-step images and text), how to make the *Transition* to the next exercise, *Precision points* to be aware of and *Common errors* to avoid. Also listed are *Modifications* for each exercise, which form an essential tool to make Pilates accessible to most people. Use them to enable you to perform an exercise safely; they also serve as building blocks to help you, in time, achieve the ideal form of the exercise. Modifications are useful when recovering from injury, or if you struggle with flexibility, are deconditioned or have a weak or poorly functioning core. Do not be at all discouraged if you need to use the Modifications, or let it put you off from continuing with your Pilates journey. Everyone needs to work within their own capabilities.

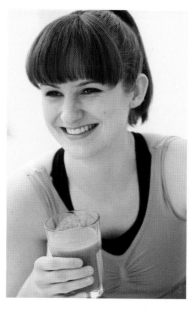

COMBINING EXERCISES WITH CLASS PRACTICE

Unfortunately there is no "quick fix" in achieving the goals that you want to attain by starting Pilates; it takes an element of motivation from the student. Joseph Pilates encouraged people to practice four times a week, even for a short time. The truth is that to feel the benefits in your body, you need to practice.

If you attend a class weekly, use this book as an adjunct and practice two or three times a week in between your classes. The emphasis is on quality: if your time is limited, ensure that what you do is of the best quality, even if it is a shorter routine, rather than doing the complete mat workout poorly. As you become more proficient you will be able to complete a longer workout in less time, but with the same level of precision. Two ten-minute workouts are provided in Chapter 8 (see pages 364–77); this is a useful practice tool whenever you are unable to dedicate a longer period of time to practicing.

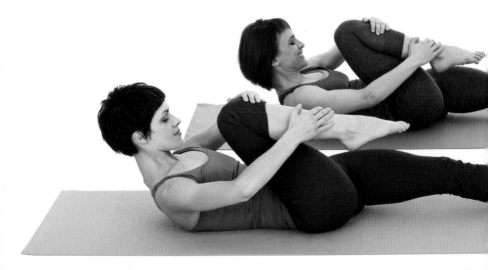

One way to complement your practice is to bring what you have learned during your workout into your everyday life. For instance, use your scoop as you go about your everyday activities; or, when you feel lifted and lengthened after your Pilates session, try to reproduce that feeling as you walk around.

EQUIPMENT

The only piece of equipment that you absolutely must have to start Pilates is a mat. Ideally your mat should be thick enough to cushion your spine and joints when rolling and exercising during your workout. A 10mm-thick mat will provide the desired amount of protection. Your mat should not slip on the floor, and your hands and feet should be able to grip the mat to avoid slipping.

You don't need specialized clothing—your clothes just need to be loose enough so that you can move freely, and they should not impede your movement. There are one or two other small pieces of equipment commonly associated with Pilates,

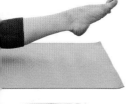

such as exercise bands, magic circles, foam rollers, small balls and gym balls, although you don't need any of these to bring Pilates into your fitness program. Some of the exercise descriptions refer to using a "block" for the *Modifications*, but this doesn't need to be a specially purchased piece of equipment; you can use a small firm cushion, a telephone directory or a rolled-up jumper.

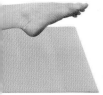

In Chapter 7, the Arm-Weight series of exercises (see pages 350–63), the text mentions using small hand-weights. These are optional; in fact, the benefits of the exercises can be gained using "self-resistance," and use of the weights simply intensifies the workout. Alternatives to hand-weights, such as small bottles filled with water, can be used instead. Just ensure that you have a steady grip on the item, to prevent injury.

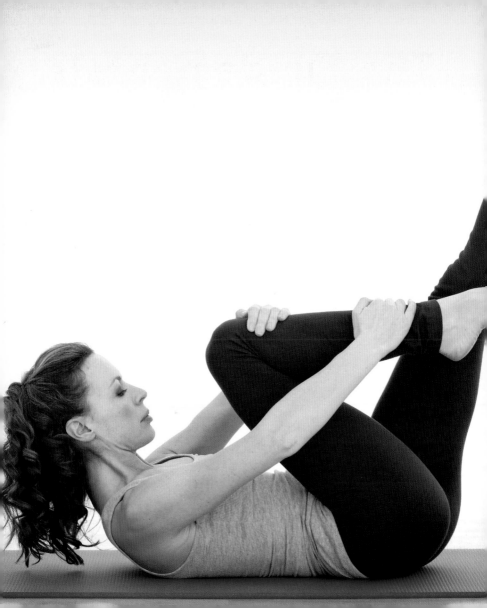

The Fundamentals

The Fundamentals teach you the basic principle of using and scooping your powerhouse to stabilize your back and pelvis, while gently imposing movement on top: "stability with mobility." They take key components of the bigger exercises and break them down into achievable parts, correcting movement patterns that may have become faulty through injury, poor posture or the stresses and strains of everyday life. The Fundamentals are a useful tool when first starting Pilates, when recovering from injury, and when bringing your attention to your body at the beginning of a session.

Imprinting

GOALS:
- ✓ Helps release muscles that are overactive, in preparation for working the correct muscles
- ✓ Enables the spine to let go, align and gently imprint itself on the mat
- ✓ Begins to bring the focus of the mind into the body

1 **Lie on your back with your knees bent and feet flat on the mat.** Turn your palms up and slide your arms out to the side, so that they rest comfortably on the mat. Your neck should be lengthened, use a block under the head if required. Inhale through your nose to expand your lungs out to the sides. Exhale and let your out-breath travel down through the spine as each of the bones releases onto the mat.

INFORMATION

NUMBER OF REPETITIONS
3–5 breaths.

VISUALIZATION The muscles in your back melt into the mat.

Breathing

GOALS: ✓ Teaches expansion of the lungs and increases their capacity

✓ Increases awareness of the breath

✓ Helps lengthen the spine onto the mat

1 **Lie on your back with your knees bent and legs together, feet flat, arms by your side.** Use a block or pillow under your head if you need to. Inhale through your nose to fill your lungs out into the ribs: to the side, to the back and to the top. Exhale completely and let the ribs soften into your centerline as your spine lengthens on the mat.

INFORMATION

NUMBER OF REPETITIONS
3–5 breaths.

VISUALIZATION Your lungs fill up like two balloons.

Iso-Abs

GOALS: ✓ Teaches how to "scoop"

1 **Lie on your back with your knees bent, feet flat and spine softly imprinted onto the mat.** Bring your hands onto your lower abdomen, with your thumbs on your navel and index fingers on your pubic bone, creating a diamond shape. Inhale, then as you exhale pull in your lower abdominals at the fingertips, in the middle of the diamond and at your navel. The muscles should hollow the abdomen, but the pelvis should stay still.

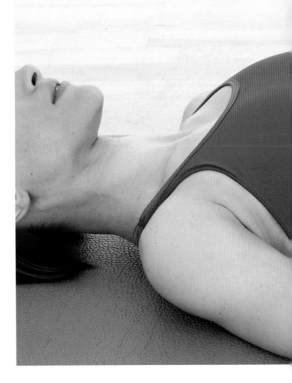

INFORMATION

NUMBER OF REPETITIONS
3–5 breaths; don't let the scoop release
between each breath.

VISUALIZATION Zip up your lower
abdomen as if you're zipping up a tight
pair of jeans.

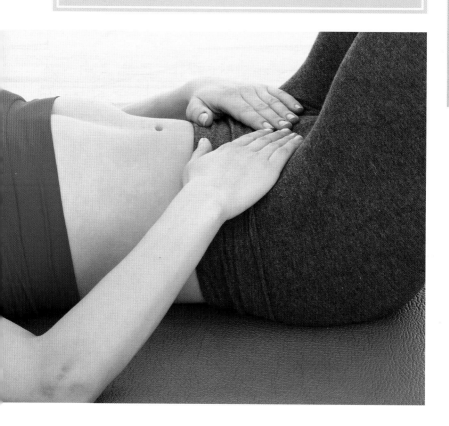

Head Nods

GOALS: ✓ Teaches how to initiate the lift of the head correctly

✓ Teaches how to separate the head from the neck

1 **Lie on your back with your knees bent and feet flat,** arms by your side.

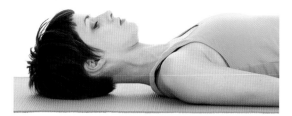

2 **Lengthen through the crown of your head,** so that the chin gently tips to the chest and the back of the neck elongates.

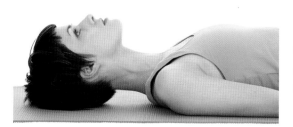

3 **Tip the chin up softly to the ceiling,** then tip it down to the chest again as the back of the neck lengthens.

INFORMATION

NUMBER OF REPETITIONS 3–5.

VISUALIZATION Pivot your head on an axle through your ears.

Neck Curls

GOALS: ✓ Teaches how to lift the head correctly using the power-house

✓ Engages the upper abdominals to help support the head during exercises where the head is up

1 **Lie on your back with your knees bent and feet flat,** arms by your side.

INFORMATION

NUMBER OF REPETITIONS 3–5.

VISUALIZATION Press your sternum and bottom rib into the mat to lift your head.

Reach through the crown of your head to lengthen your neck, tip your chin to your chest and lift your head to look at your navel, sliding the ribs into the waist as you roll your head up. Keep your shoulders broad and your chest open.

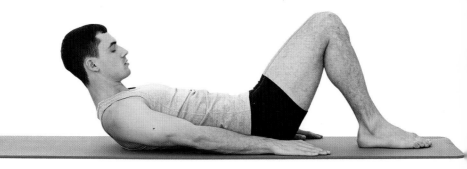

Lengthen through the crown of your head to roll back down. Don't let your chin poke to the ceiling at any time. Your face, jaw and throat should stay soft.

Clock

GOALS: ✓ Mobilizes the pelvis on the lumbar spine at the lower back, and vice versa

✓ Optimizes finding the neutral or mid-position of the pelvis

✓ Uses the abdominal muscles in a small movement

1 **Lie on your back with your knees bent and feet flat.** Imagine that you have a clock face on your lower abdomen: 12 o'clock is at your navel and 6 o'clock is at your pubic bone.

INFORMATION

NUMBER OF REPETITIONS 3–5.

VISUALIZATION Use the movement in your pelvis to roll a marble between the 12 o'clock and 6 o'clock positions on the clock face.

2 **Using your abdominals, roll the 6 o'clock position to the 12 o'clock position,** so that your tailbone curls under.

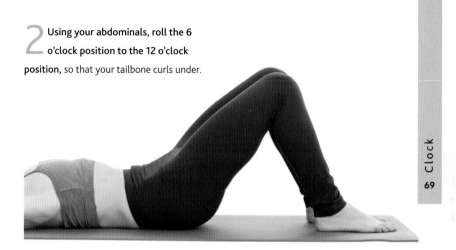

3 **Lengthen your pubic bone away from your navel (6 o'clock away from 12 o'clock),** so that your tailbone touches the mat and there is daylight between the mat and your lower back.

Ribcage Arms

GOALS:
- ✓ Teaches the connection between the shoulders and the trunk, and how to stabilize the shoulder blades on the trunk
- ✓ Teaches how to work the arms in the joint, rather than letting the shoulders slide up to the ears
- ✓ Engages the upper part of the abdominals as they attach to the ribs

1 Lie on your back with your knees bent and feet flat. Take your hands to the ceiling, with your shoulder blades and ribs imprinted on the mat.

INFORMATION

NUMBER OF REPETITIONS 3–5.

VISUALIZATION The back of your ribs are set in wet sand. The front of your ribs are knitted together.

2 **Exhale and float your arms back to reach your fingers behind you.** The back of your ribs and your spine should stay in contact with the mat; the front of the ribs should stay funnelled into your waist. Then inhale and float your arms back to the starting position.

Knee Folds

GOALS: ✓ Trains how to stabilize the back and pelvis, using the powerhouse while moving a leg

✓ Teaches how to move the legs separately from the pelvis, rather than in a rigid "block"

✓ Challenges the scoop

1 **Lie on your back with your knees bent and feet flat.** Scoop your powerhouse in and up, then float the right knee up over the right hip, maintaining the imprint of your spine and your pelvis in the mid-position. Return your foot to the mat, then repeat with the left leg. Lift your legs alternately, keeping your tailbone on the mat and each knee in line with the hip and shoulder.

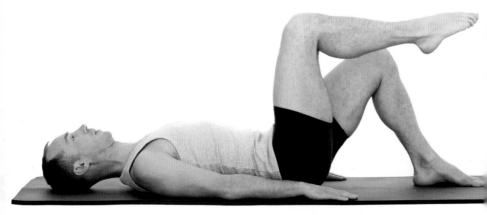

INFORMATION

NUMBER OF REPETITIONS
3–5 on each leg.

VISUALIZATION Balance a saucer of milk on your stomach; don't let your back or stomach muscles shift, or the milk will spill.

2 **To progress: as you lower one foot to the mat,** lift the other, so that your legs pass each other in space and both feet are momentarily off the mat. Your spine must stay imprinted on the mat, and your abdominals engaged and hollowed.

Knee Spreads

GOALS: ✓ Stabilizes the pelvis while moving a leg

✓ Challenges the scoop

✓ Trains stability and control at the hips and pelvis

✓ Improves the mobility of the hip joint

1 Lie on your back with your knees bent and feet flat.

INFORMATION

NUMBER OF REPETITIONS
3–5 on each leg.

VISUALIZATION Your legs open like
the petals of a flower.

2 **Scoop your powerhouse,** then keep
your left knee facing the ceiling and
lower your right knee out to the side, without your pelvis shifting. Bring the right
knee back to the center with control, then
repeat with the left leg.

Knee Sways

GOALS:
- ✓ Mobilizes the spine through rotation
- ✓ Challenges the oblique abdominal muscles
- ✓ Lengthens the muscles down each side of the back and legs

1 Lie on your back with your knees bent and feet flat.

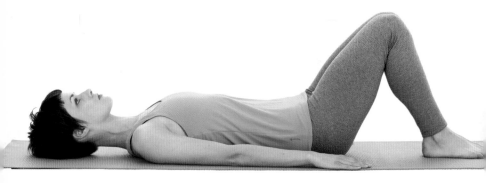

INFORMATION

NUMBER OF REPETITIONS
3–5 each way.

VISUALIZATION Your abdominals winch your legs back to the center.

2 **Scoop your abdominals in and up, keeping your feet flat on the mat, and lower your knees toward the mat.** The pelvis should lift as the legs lower, but the ribs and shoulder should stay imprinted on the mat to create a stretch through the waist, lower back and outside of the hip. Scoop your pelvis to use your abdominals to bring your legs back to the center, then repeat to the other side.

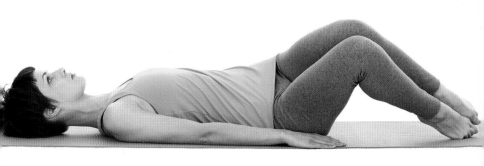

Leg Slides

GOALS: ✓ Trains stability of the pelvis and lower back while the leg
moves

✓ Teaches how to move the legs from the powerhouse,
not the thigh muscles

1 Lie on your back with your
knees bent and feet flat.

INFORMATION

NUMBER OF REPETITIONS
3–5 on each leg.

VISUALIZATION Your heel is sliding
effortlessly on glass.

2 **Scoop your abdominals and press your right heel into the mat,** then slide your right leg out along the mat to lengthen out of your hip.

3 **Your knee should stay in line with your hip and shoulder.** Pulling your abdominals in deeper, slide your heel back in to the starting position, with the foot flat. Repeat with the other leg.

Flight

GOALS: ✓ Increases awareness of where the shoulder blades
should sit on the upper back
✓ Works the muscles of the upper back
✓ Encourages the big muscles that elevate the shoulders
to the ears to relax and stretch
✓ Opens the front of the chest

1 **Lie on your front with your
forehead on the mat,** arms by
your side and palms facing the ceiling.

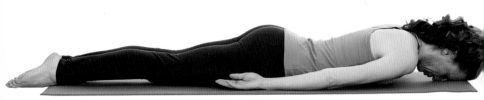

INFORMATION

NUMBER OF REPETITIONS 3–5.

VISUALIZATION As you take your shoulder blades to the ceiling, crack a walnut between them.

2 **Scoop, take your shoulders up to your ears, pull your shoulder blades to the ceiling and slide them down your back.** Your head and sternum should lengthen slightly off the mat.

Reach your fingers long toward the end of the mat. Turn your palms down to the mat, then back to the ceiling, and lower your chest, shoulders and head gently back onto the mat.

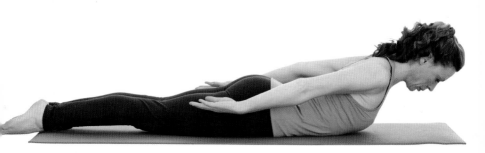

Goalpost Arms

GOALS:
- ✓ Increases awareness of where the shoulder blades should sit on the upper back
- ✓ Works the muscles of the upper back
- ✓ Encourages the big muscles that elevate the shoulders to the ears to relax and stretch
- ✓ Opens the front of the chest
- ✓ Teaches how to stabilize the shoulder blades onto the back and ribs

1 **Lie on your front with your arms out at shoulder level, your elbows at a 90° angle and your palms flat on the mat.** Your legs are hip-width apart.

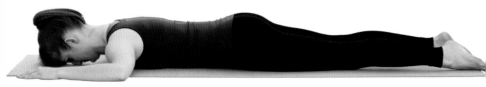

INFORMATION

NUMBER OF REPETITIONS 3–5.

CAUTIONS For rotator-cuff and other shoulder problems, omit this exercise.

VISUALIZATION Your shoulder blades slide into your back pockets.

2 **Press your elbows into the mat to lift your forearms and hands to the ceiling.** Your head should float up too. Initiate the movement by sliding your shoulder blades down your back. Lengthen down to return to the mat.

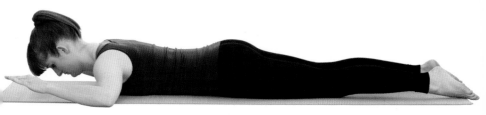

Beginner's Program

"... beginning with the introductory lesson, each succeeding exercise should be mastered before proceeding progressively with the following exercises." JOSEPH PILATES

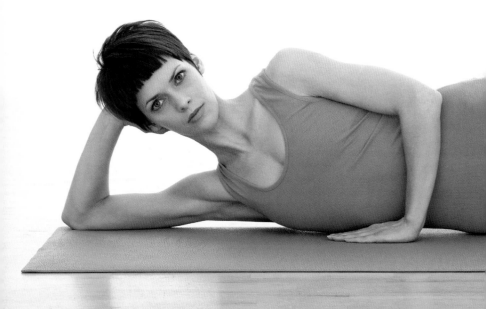

The Beginner's Program introduces your body to moving, using the Pilates principles. The main focus of the beginner's workout is to teach you to use the powerhouse to stabilize your lower back and pelvis during movement, following the Pilates principles of control and centering. The Beginner's Program offers numerous Modifications to the exercises to make Pilates accessible, regardless of your starting point.

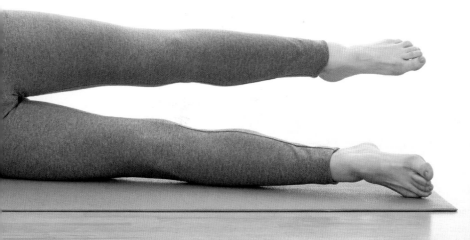

The Hundred

GOALS: ✓ Teaches how to engage the powerhouse and maintain it
for the duration of the exercise

✓ Helps you to breathe while the powerhouse is engaged

✓ Warms up the powerhouse

1 **Lie on your back with your knees bent, feet flat, and scoop your powerhouse in and up.** Your abdominals will be pulled in and active, so that your back is softly imprinted on the mat from your tailbone to the crown of your head.

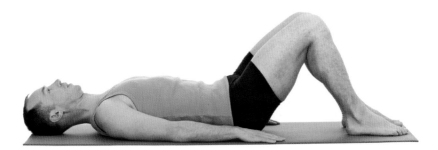

2 **Lift one knee at a time, so that your knees are over your hips** and your legs are bent at a 90° angle in the tabletop position. Your legs should be pressed together.

3 **Lift your chin to your chest and simultaneously lift your hands to hip height, reaching long through your fingertips.** Breathe in for a count of 5, pumping your arms 6–8 inches (15–20 cm).

Then breathe out for a count of 5, all the time pumping your arms 6–8 inches (15–20 cm). Your arms should pump to the rhythm of your breath: 5 pumps for the in-breath, 5 pumps for the out-breath.

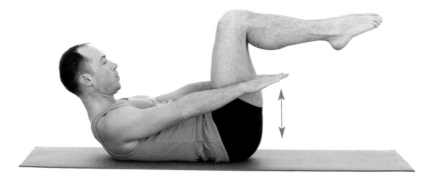

MODIFICATIONS

If the exercise pulls on your neck,
use a block under your head; either
keep the pumps of the arms small
or omit pumping the arms.

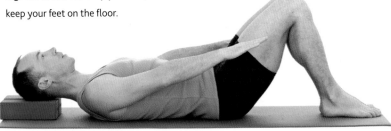

> **TRANSITION** Bring your knees in to your
> chest, chin to chest, and roll up in one, to
> come into sitting for the Roll Down.

**If you are unable to maintain the
imprint of your spine when your
legs are in the tabletop position,**
keep your feet on the floor.

COMMON ERRORS

- Losing the position of the head, so that it falls back and the neck is strained
- The abdominals popping so that they bulge and the imprint of the spine on the mat is lost
- The shoulder blades sliding up to the ears, and losing the connection with the ribs at the back

INFORMATION

NUMBER OF REPETITIONS Start with 20–30 pumps, 2–3 breaths; progress to 100 pumps, 10 breaths.

CAUTIONS If you experience neck strain, lower your head and use a block, as in the Modifications (see left). For back problems and weak abdominals, ensure there is no strain in the back—if there is, place your feet on the mat. For back or neck issues, follow the Modifications and gradually progress so that you can get your legs into the tabletop position and your head up.

VISUALIZATION Fill your lungs out to the sides.

PRECISION POINTS

- The wrists are kept strong; the fingers reach long.
- The chin stays in to the chest, with the back of the neck lengthened.
- The ribs are funnelled in.
- The shoulder blades slide down the back.
- The spine stays imprinted on the mat.
- The legs stay pressed together in the centerline.

Roll Down

1 **Sit up with your knees bent, feet flat on the floor and legs hip-width apart.** Hold behind your thighs with both hands, with your elbows lifted and shoulders down. Your powerhouse is pulled in and up.

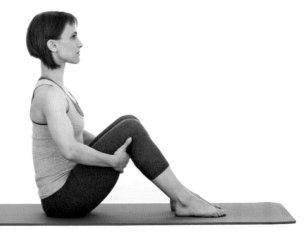

2 **Initiate the move from the base of your spine.** Engage your backside muscles and tilt your pelvis back, so that you "tuck your tail under." Tilt your chin down to look at your navel.

3 **As you roll back, imprint one vertebra at a time into the mat,** using your abdominal muscles to help place each bone as you articulate through the C-curve. When your elbows are straight, pull your powerhouse in deeper, and begin to curl back up to the starting position.

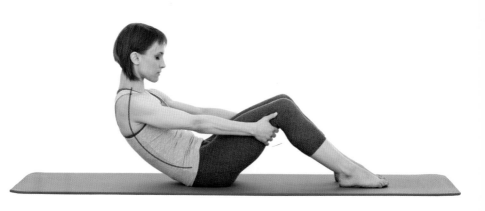

TRANSITION Roll down to the mat
ready for One-Leg Circles.

MODIFICATIONS

If your feet don't go flat onto the mat,
keep them flexed. Prepare for the exercise
by just tucking your tail under, rather than
starting to roll back.

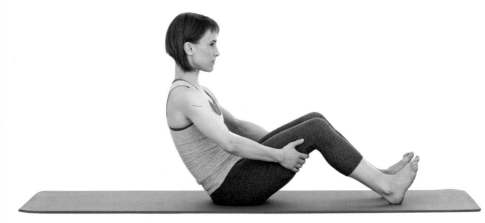

COMMON ERRORS

- Chin poking out
- Losing the connection of the abdominals and ribs, leading to the abdominals bulging
- Being unable to find the C-curve and lowering down with a flat back
- Feet lifting off the mat

INFORMATION

NUMBER OF REPETITIONS 4.

CAUTIONS If you have lower back pain proceed with caution, or omit the exercise. If you have a sore or painful coccyx you may want to omit this exercise.

VISUALIZATION Pizza-wheel your spine down onto the mat.

PRECISION POINTS

- The abdominals are kept lifted, with your navel in to your spine, to help articulation of the spine.
- The powerhouse (not your arms) is used to bring you back up.
- The descent is controlled; do not flop back!
- The shoulders should remain down and the elbows out.

One-Leg Circles

GOALS: ✓ Teaches how to stabilize the hips and pelvis, while
moving the leg separately from the body
✓ Builds flexibility of the hamstrings
✓ Strengthens the hip muscles

1 **Lie on the mat, bend your knees
and place your feet firmly on the
mat**; imprint your spine softly onto the
mat. Bend your right knee in to your
chest, then lengthen the leg toward the
ceiling, with a slight turn-out, into the
Pilates stance (see page 34).

2 **Inhale and move your right leg across your body to the opposite hip,** but do not let your right hip lift off the mat.

3 **To form the circle,** take your leg down a small distance along the centerline and then over to the side, in line with the right shoulder.

4 Exhale and finish the circle, bringing the leg back to the starting position. On completing 5 repetitions, reverse the circles. Then bring your right knee in to the chest and lower your foot to the floor. Change legs and repeat with the left leg.

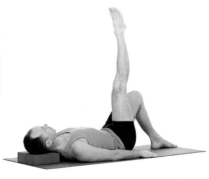

TRANSITION Bring your knees in to your chest, holding them behind the thighs, and bring chin to chest. Roll up in one movement, bringing yourself forward on the mat for Rolling Like a Ball.

MODIFICATIONS

If your neck and/or shoulders are tight, place your head on a block.

If your hamstrings are tight, use a soft bend in the elevated leg to enable you to maintain the imprint of your spine and tailbone on the mat while you move your leg.

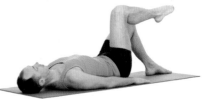

COMMON ERRORS

- Bracing with the head, neck and shoulders, which can strain the neck
- The belly popping, and losing the imprint of the spine, with the back arching and the pelvis tipping forward and back and from side to side
- Curling the tail off the mat

INFORMATION

NUMBER OF REPETITIONS 5 each way, on each leg.

CAUTIONS For neck problems, use a block under the head. For back problems, maintain the imprint of your spine on the mat by either bending your knee or using a band, if required. If your hip clicks, either keep your knee bent or omit the exercise.

VISUALIZATION Draw perfect small circles on the ceiling. Visualize a line drawn through your center, from your crown to your heels, and work to the center.

PRECISION POINTS
- The back of the neck is kept lengthened.
- The "box" is kept square and work is done within the "frame."
- Both hips are kept firmly plugged onto the mat, so that the pelvis does not shift.
- The spine stays imprinted into the mat.

Rolling Like a Ball

GOALS:
- ✓ Massages the spine
- ✓ Teaches control
- ✓ Trains the abdominals
- ✓ Teaches how to work toward your centerline

1 **Sit at the front of the mat with your knees bent.** Lift one foot at a time, so that you balance on your sitting bones, and hold behind the thighs with your hands, with your elbows high and wide. Slide your shoulders down your back, and bring your chin to your chest. You are now in your starting position,

feeling balanced on your sit-bones, with your tummy muscles helping to keep you from falling back. You should feel as if your spine is in the shape of a C, but lifted by your abdominals.

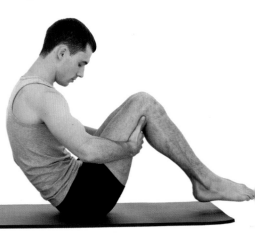

2 **Inhale, pull your abdominals in,** and control your descent as you roll backward, with your tailbone tucked under. Keep your shape!

3 **Exhale and use your abdominals— *not* your arms—to roll back up.** Find your balance on your sit-bones at the top of the roll, using your powerhouse to prevent a wobble!

TRANSITION Place your feet on the floor, take your bottom back and roll down to the mat for the Single Leg Stretch.

If you are unable to come back up without straining, then just balance where you are, or rock in the balance position, using your abdominals.

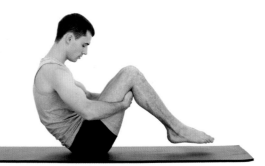

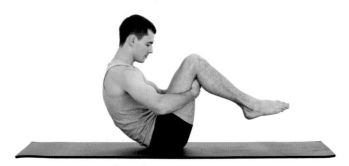

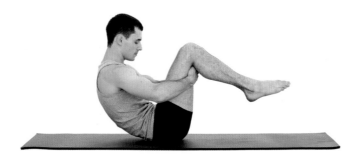

COMMON ERRORS

- Rolling onto your neck
- Lifting the shoulders to the ears
- Using the movement of your arms and shoulders to help you come up
- Throwing the feet forward
- Bringing the chin away from the chest, and throwing the head around

INFORMATION

NUMBER OF REPETITIONS 6–8.

CAUTIONS For osteoporosis, omit any rolling exercises if you have bone-density problems more severe than osteopenia (a condition in which bone density is lower than normal, often seen as a precursor to osteoporosis). If you have significant scoliosis, omit this exercise. For back problems, proceed with caution; if you have disc problems, omit this exercise. If you have knee problems, be mindful of how your knees are feeling.

VISUALIZATION Rock in a rocking chair! Rock back until you are going to tip over, then rock back up.

PRECISION POINTS

- It is important to keep your shape.
- The abdominals, not the arms, are used to roll you up. Rolling is to the tip of the shoulder blades only.
- The lower back is kept lifted into the C-curve throughout.

Abdominal Five Series: Single Leg Stretch

GOALS: ✓ Works the abdominals

✓ Teaches alignment and how to work strongly along the centerline

✓ The powerhouse stabilizes the trunk on the mat and keeps it still while the limbs move

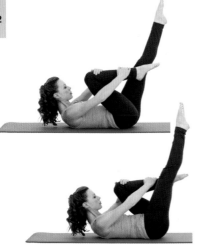

TRANSITION Lower your head to rest your neck. Bring your knees in to your chest and hold your ankles, ready for the Double Leg Stretch.

1 **Lie in the center of your mat, with both knees drawn into your chest and chin to chest, with your eyes on your navel.** Anchor your middle onto the mat by scooping your abdominals. Pull your right knee into the chest, with your right hand on the ankle and left hand on the right knee. Lengthen your left leg to the ceiling. Your elbows should be high and wide, with the shoulders soft and down.

2 **Inhale and change legs; hug your left knee in to your chest, in line with your left shoulder;** reach your right leg long and strong to the ceiling, in line with your centerline, in the Pilates stance. Exhale and change legs, keeping strongly centered, with your spine imprinted from the tailbone to the base of your shoulder blades.

MODIFICATIONS

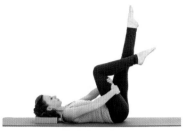

If you have knee problems, hold behind the thigh rather than on the knee. Use a block if you have a fragile neck.

For back problems or weak abdominals, bend your knees with your feet flat on the floor; chin to your chest; lift one knee, hug it in to your chest; lower it slowly and change legs, alternating legs one at a time.

COMMON ERRORS

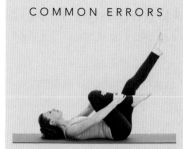

- Losing the imprint of your spine, causing the trunk to rock from side to side
- Losing the midline, with the legs wandering out to the side, away from the centerline
- The abdominals bulging during the switch of the legs
- The shoulders creeping up toward the ears

INFORMATION

NUMBER OF REPETITIONS Start with 3 for each leg, then progress to 6; the maximum number of repetitions is 10.

CAUTIONS For knee, neck and back issues, refer to the Modifications.

VISUALIZATION Your shoulders and hips form the corners of a box, with a line through the center; all movement glides along the line and the box stays firm.

PRECISION POINTS
- The abdominals stay lifted through-out.
- Keep the box square.
- The legs lengthen along the centerline.
- Keep the ribs pulled in, with the tops of the shoulders lifted off the mat and the eyes locked into your navel.

Abdominal Five Series: Double Leg Stretch

1 **Lie on your back in the center of the mat and place your hands as close to your ankles as the length of your arms allows.** Lift your chin to your chest using your powerhouse, with your eyes toward your navel and your knees slightly apart.

Your heels should be close to your bottom and your elbows lifted, with the tips of your shoulder blades on the mat. Draw in your powerhouse to ensure you are firmly imprinted on the mat, from your tailbone to the tips of your shoulder blades.

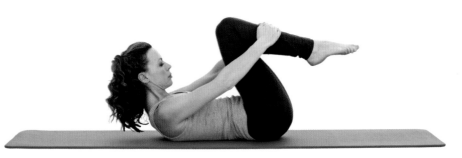

2 **Inhale and take your arms up by your ears, and your legs toward the ceiling at a 90° angle, in the Pilates stance.** Your head should stay lifted and does not move, and your abdominals should stay scooped, with your front ribs sliding toward your navel.

3 **Exhale and begin to circle your arms** round to your sides.

4 **Pull your knees in from the abdominals,** as you hug your legs back into the starting position.

> **TRANSITION** Pull your knees in tighter to your chest and roll up to a sitting position for the Spine Stretch Forward.

MODIFICATIONS

For a weak lower back, weak abdominals or difficulty in maintaining the imprint of your spine, as you reach your limbs away take your legs to the tabletop position, with your hips and knees at a 90° angle and your arms toward the ceiling.

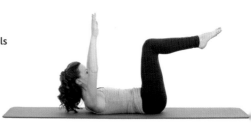

For neck problems, keep your head on a block and only take your legs to the tabletop position, with your arms toward the ceiling.

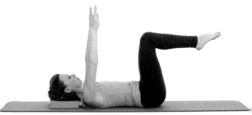

COMMON ERRORS

- Chin poking to the ceiling
- The lower back arching off the mat
- Losing the imprint of your tailbone on the mat
- Shoulders elevating to the ears

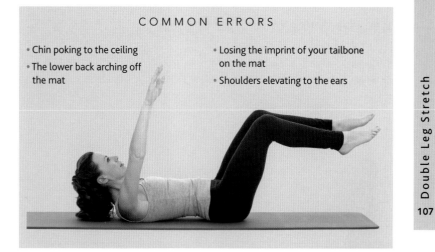

INFORMATION

NUMBER OF REPETITIONS 6.

CAUTIONS For knee pain, take your hands behind your thighs. For shoulder pain, keep the movement of the arms smaller by lifting your arms directly to the ceiling, avoid circling the arms and just lower directly to bring the hands to the ankles.

VISUALIZATION Fill the lungs as you stretch; squeeze the air out as you hug.

PRECISION POINTS

- Your tailbone stays on the mat when hugging the knees.
- The legs work to the centerline as you lengthen them away.
- The ribs stay imprinted on the mat throughout, and the shoulders stay engaged.
- The spine lengthens on the mat, from the tailbone to the tips of the shoulder blades.

Spine Stretch Forward

GOALS:
✓ Provides a stretch to the hamstrings and moves the individual vertebra of the spine

✓ Brings you up against gravity and starts to train the powerhouse to work in an upright position

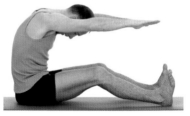

1 **Sit tall on the mat with your legs apart—just wider than your shoulders—and knees slightly bent.** Grow the spine tall, lift your arms to shoulder height and extend them forward. When you have a sense of being "lifted" and sitting tall by using your powerhouse and a lengthened spine, then you have achieved a good set-up position.

2 **Exhale and bring your chin to your chest; place your head between your arms as you curl down, rounding your upper back.** Continue curling down as your navel pulls deeply into your spine. Create a deep stretch as your hands reach forward and your powerhouse pulls into the lower back to stretch it out further; continue to flex the feet. Squeeze all the air out of your lungs, then inhale and use your abdominals to roll back up and sit tall, with your shoulders directly over your hips.

TRANSITION Stay in the seated position, with your spine lifted and knees softly bent; take your arms out to the sides, within the line of your vision, for Saw.

MODIFICATIONS

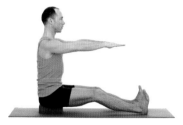

For tight hamstrings and a stiff lower back, maintain the soft knee bend and sit on a block—use a size that enables you to sit with your shoulders over your hips, without straining.

For shoulder problems, slide your hands along the mat inside your legs.

COMMON ERRORS

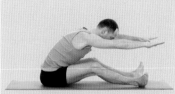

- Losing the energy in the legs, so that the feet aren't flexed and the knees roll inward
- Leading with the chin so that the shoulders lift up to the ears and the arms turn in
- Bending at the hips, rather than using the powerhouse to lift the spine

INFORMATION

NUMBER OF REPETITIONS 5.

CAUTIONS If your lower back feels tight, make the movement smaller and build up to the bigger stretch. For lower back and shoulder problems, follow the Modifications.

VISUALIZATION Roll away from an imaginary wall behind you to roll down; to come up, place one vertebra at a time up against that imaginary wall.

PRECISION POINTS
- Keep the legs active so that your toes and knees stay facing the ceiling.
- A lifted "round" in the spine should be created, not a flat back.
- The spine is stacked to roll back up; don't come up in one movement, with a flat back.
- An active backside is maintained, to keep you lifted throughout the move.

Saw

GOALS: ✔ Works the spine's range of motion into rotation, supported by a strong center
✔ Begins to train the stamina of the powerhouse in a position against gravity

1 **Sit on the mat with your feet just wider than the mat and your knees softly bent.** Using your powerhouse and backside muscles, lift out of your hips and lengthen your spine through the crown of your head. Reach your arms out to the sides, but still within your vision. It is important to achieve a feeling of being tall and lifted in the sitting position, with both sides of your waist lengthened, but your shoulders down.

2 **Inhale and lift your spine from your powerhouse, as you twist at the waist to the right.** Your buttocks should be working to anchor your hips into the mat.

3 **Exhale and keep the C-curve as you reach your left little finger past your right little toe;** your right hand reaches up and back, and your ear moves toward your knee. Deepen the exhale as you reach for a count of 1, 2 and then even further for 3. Inhale and pull your abdominals in to grow tall, then twist to the left and repeat the action.

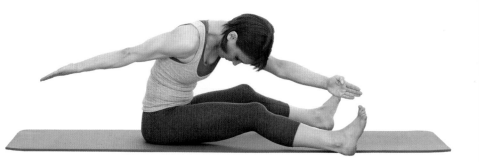

TRANSITION Bring your arms and legs together, bend your knees and roll down and onto your right side for the Side Kick series.

MODIFICATIONS

For tight hamstrings or lower back, sit on a block to lift your hips.

COMMON ERRORS

- The knees rolling inward, if the alignment is lost at the hips
- The arms swinging around—keep them in line with the shoulders
- Not keeping the buttocks anchored into the mat as you reach
- Flopping from the hips, rather than lifting into the C-curve

INFORMATION

NUMBER OF REPETITIONS 3.

CAUTIONS If you have restrictions in your shoulders, follow the Modifications, or omit the exercise. For back difficulties, particularly disc problems, be aware of how your back will cope with the combination of twist and bend; either use the Modifications or omit this exercise until the issue has resolved sufficiently to enable you to proceed.

VISUALIZATION Your hips and legs are set in wet cement; the lift and twist come from above.

PRECISION POINTS

- The hips stay static on the mat; don't let the buttocks lift as you reach.
- Both heels stay level, with the knees facing the ceiling.
- The spine is articulated to sit up out of the C-curve—don't come up with a flat back.
- Lifting is used to decompress the spine as you twist.
- The eyes follow the hand as it moves behind.
- Keep your shoulders sliding down your back.

Side Kick Series: Front/Back

✓ Tones, lengthens and strengthens the legs, hips and abdominals

✓ Creates flexibility in the hamstrings

✓ Trains core stability and balance in a different position

1 **Lie on your side, in line with the back edge of the mat.** Support yourself on your elbow, with your head on your hand, keeping the back of your neck long. Your top hand is your stabilizing one: place it flat on the mat with the fingers turned to your face and your elbow bent and flush to the

hip. Your body has now created a long, strong line along the back of the mat; ensure your powerhouse is active, lifting the waist so that you have a sense that your abdominals are defying gravity, to prevent your stomach falling forward onto the mat.

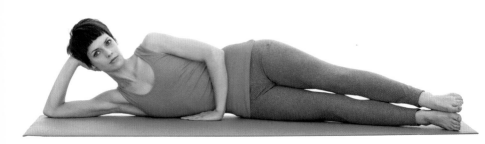

2 Bring your legs forward, so that your feet are at the front corner of the mat or at a 45° angle, with the bend in your hips and your top hand on the mat; you should feel stable and secure enough to allow you to move the top leg freely.

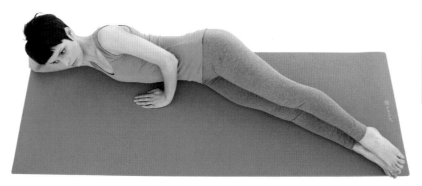

3 Inhale and lift the top leg to hip height; kick forward, keeping your hips and shoulders stacked and your top leg parallel with the floor.

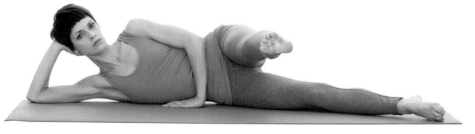

4 **Take your top leg back, reaching it behind the hip with a straight knee and active seat muscles.** Breathe naturally, then kick forward and kick back again with a long leg.

TRANSITION Bring your top heel to your bottom heel, with a slight turn toward the ceiling of the knee on your top leg, ready for Up/Down.

MODIFICATIONS

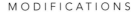

For neck or shoulder problems, rest your head on a block, so that your neck remains in line with the rest of your spine and your bottom arm is extended forward. Experiment with the size of block to get the correct one for you. The Side Kick series is repeated on both sides of the body, so ensure you treat both sides the same.

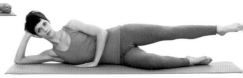

For weak abdominals and poor balance, bend your bottom leg until you gain strength, so that you can work toward getting the bottom leg straight. For hip problems, including hip replacements, keep the movement smaller.

COMMON ERRORS

- Losing the box, so that the shoulders and hips rock back and forth
- Using momentum, so that the top leg moves without control

- Turning the head to look at the feet, so that the spine bends

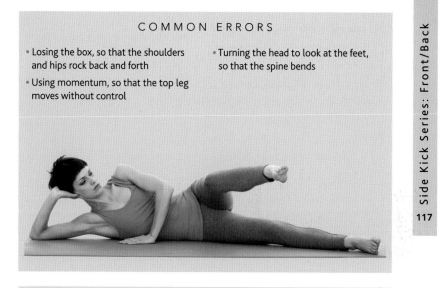

INFORMATION

NUMBER OF REPETITIONS 5.

CAUTIONS For hip problems, including hip replacements and hips that "clunk," keep the movement smaller and work with active seat muscles. For neck and shoulder problems, follow the Modifications.

VISUALIZATION Balance a cup and saucer on your shoulder and hip—don't let it rattle or spill!

PRECISION POINTS

- The eyes stay forward; the spine stays long from crown to tail.
- The hips and shoulders remain stacked.
- The top leg stays parallel to the floor, and remains long and strong.

Side Kick Series: Up/Down

GOALS:
- ✓ Tones, lengthens and strengthens the legs, hips and abdominals
- ✓ Adds flexibility of the inner thigh
- ✓ Begins to challenge stability and balance

1 **Lie on your side, with your head on one hand and the other hand on the mat in front.** You should be lined up at the back of your mat, with your legs at a 45° angle. Your top heel should be in contact with your bottom heel, with your top leg slightly turned out.

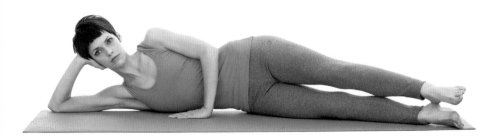

2 **Inhale and lift your top leg straight toward the ceiling,** without the hips and pelvis changing their alignment.

3 **To lower the leg,** exhale and resist your own movement as you reach the leg long.

TRANSITION Return to the starting position for Inner Thigh Lifts and Circles.

For neck and shoulder problems, place a
block under your head, ensuring it is of the
correct height so that your neck doesn't
feel any strain.

For weak abdominals and poor balance, bend
your bottom leg until you gain strength, so that
you can work toward getting the bottom leg
straight. For hip problems, including hip
replacements, keep the movement smaller.

COMMON ERRORS

- Top hip rolling back as the leg lifts
- The knee turning in

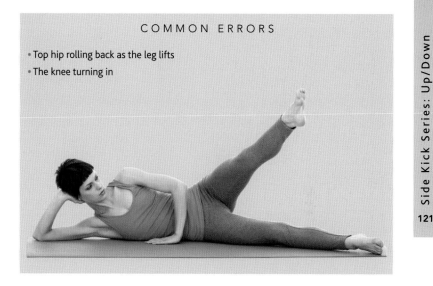

INFORMATION

NUMBER OF REPETITIONS 5.

CAUTIONS For hip problems, including hip replacements and hips that "clunk," keep the movement smaller and work with active seat muscles. For neck and shoulder problems, follow the Modifications.

VISUALIZATION Paint an arc in the air as you reach your leg up and down.

PRECISION POINTS
- Keep the top hip directly over the bottom hip.
- The neck stays long.
- The only thing that moves is the kicking leg!
- The abdominals stay scooped in and up—don't let them sink forward onto the mat.

Side Kick Series: Inner Thigh Lifts and Circles

GOALS: ✓ Brings in the opportunity to train muscle balance by working the inside of the thigh

✓ Stretches out the hip and buttock of the leg that has just worked

1 **Lie on your side on the mat, with your head in your hand; bend the top knee and place the foot flat on the floor, with your knee facing the ceiling.** Hold the ankle, bringing your hand behind the calf and wrapping it around the ankle.

Your spine should feel lengthened, despite the top hip and leg being bent; keep looking at a point directly in front of you, which will help to keep the spine from bending. Check that your spine is still parallel with the straight edge of the mat.

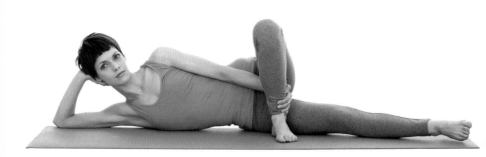

2 **Breathe naturally and lift your lower leg from the hip; the knee should stay straight.** You should feel the effort and work on the inner thigh as you lift the lower leg.

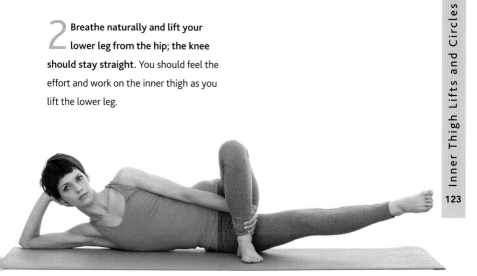

3 **Reach the leg long to lower it, but not to touch the mat.** To work the inner thigh harder, lift and then lift again, before lowering the leg.

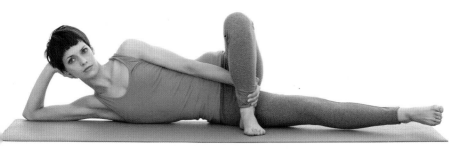

4 **After completing the last lift,** keep your leg at hip height and circle it forward 5–8 times, then reverse the action.

TRANSITION Turn to the other side to work the other leg, setting yourself up in line with the back of the mat to get into the starting position. After you have worked both sides, bring the legs together, then bend both knees and come up to a sitting position for Seal.

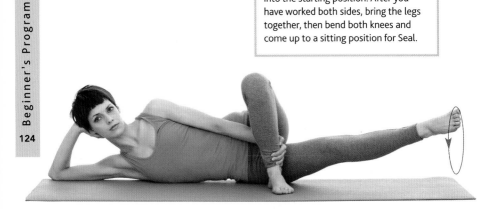

MODIFICATIONS

For neck or shoulder problems, support your head on a block and extend your arm out in front of you.

For tight knees and hips, place your bent top knee on the floor in front of you.

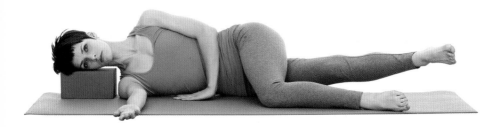

COMMON ERRORS

- Losing the work in the leg, so that the knee bends and the ankle inverts

- The top hip falling back as the vertical alignment is lost

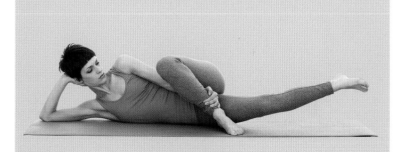

INFORMATION

NUMBER OF REPETITIONS 5.

CAUTIONS Follow the Modifications if you are unable to place the foot flat in front of you without straining the knee or hip joint. For neck issues, follow the Modifications.

VISUALIZATION Balance a teacup on the inside of your knee—don't let it rattle or spill a drop!

PRECISION POINTS

- The chest is kept open, and the eyes forward.
- The spine is lengthened from crown to tail.
- The moving leg is lengthened throughout.
- The work is from the hip; the inside of the knee faces the ceiling.
- Scooping is maintained, in and up— don't let the abdominals sink forward onto the mat.

Seal

GOALS:

✓ Opens the hips and massages the spine

✓ Trains your core to aid balance at the beginning of the move, and to control it throughout the movement

✓ Works the powerhouse

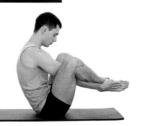

1 **Sit at the end of the mat and pull your heels in toward you.** With palms together, move your hands between your legs and place round your ankles. Scoop your powerhouse to tip back on your sit-bones and balance with feet off the mat. Press your elbows out as your knees press in. To prevent falling backward, your scoop should be pulled into your C-curve. Your arms and legs should actively work against one another to help balance; shoulder blades should be down your back. Now clap your feet together three times; move your legs from the hips, not the ankles.

2 **Inhale and use your abdominals to start rolling back, letting your tailbone tuck under as you roll.** Roll back to the tips of your shoulder blades.

3 **Exhale and, using control, roll up straight back to the starting position.** Balance, then clap your feet together three times.

TRANSITION Come up to a standing position; you have now completed the Beginner's Program.

MODIFICATIONS

For a tight lower back or vulnerable wrists and elbows, hold the legs behind the thighs.

COMMON ERRORS

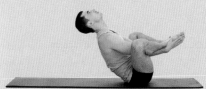

- Throwing the head back to start the roll
- Losing the frame so that the knees fall outward
- Using momentum to roll down and up, rather than exerting control
- The feet going too far and hitting the mat when you roll up
- The head and neck hitting the mat as you roll back

INFORMATION

NUMBER OF REPETITIONS 6.

CAUTIONS Omit if you have disc problems or osteoporosis, due to the flexion of the spine. Proceed with care if you have previously had a hip replacement; your hip and pelvic muscles need to have some strength to support the joint before attempting this exercise. For weak wrists and elbows, proceed with caution and follow the Modifications if necessary.

VISUALIZATION Rock like a rocking chair.

PRECISION POINTS
- The elbows and knees work in opposition: the elbows press out, the knees in.
- Keep your eyes on your center and your chin in as you roll, to keep the shape.
- Use the exhale and a deep scoop to help you roll up.

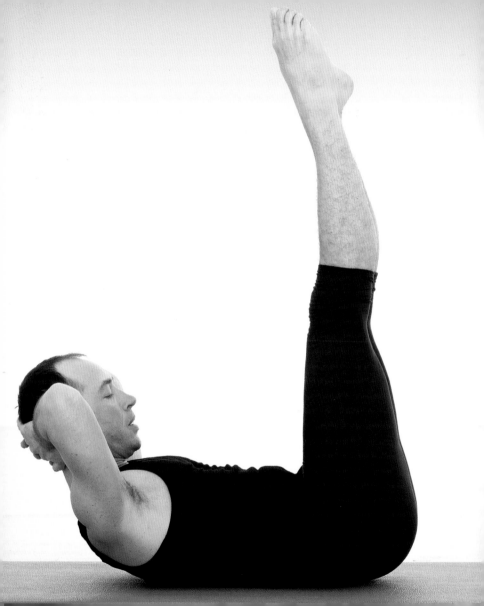

Intermediate Program

The Beginner's Program (see pages 84–127) introduced the basic moves, with a focus on control and centering. Now the Intermediate Program challenges you to start moving with flow, greater precision and concentration, getting your breath working with the exercise. The additional exercises in this workout are more demanding.

The Hundred

GOALS: ✓ Begins to challenge the stamina of the powerhouse and strengthens it

✓ Connects the breath to the powerhouse

✓ Acts as a warm-up to get the circulation going

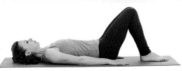

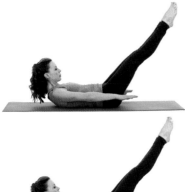

1 **Lie on your back with your knees bent**, so your powerhouse is engaged, but your spine has let go onto the mat.

2 **Scoop your powerhouse in and up and lift your legs one at a time, bending them at right-angles so that they are in tabletop position.** Simultaneously lift your chin to your chest and your hands to hip height; reach through your fingers as your shoulders slide down your back. Then lengthen your legs out to 45°, in the Pilates stance.

3 **Breathe in for 5 beats,** pumping your arms vigorously 6–8 in (15–20 cm). Breathe out for 5 beats, all the time pumping the arms 6–8 in (15–20 cm). The breath builds to the count of 5, and exhales to the count of 5.

TRANSITION Bend your knees to your chest; lower your head, then feet to the floor. Lengthen your legs and reach to the ceiling ready for Roll Up.

MODIFICATIONS

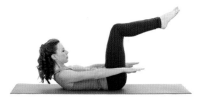

If you are unable to keep your spine imprinted on the mat for the duration of the exercise, bend your knees and keep your legs in a tabletop position. Lower your head if you feel strain in your neck, and keep your arms still.

COMMON ERRORS

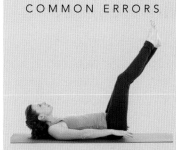

- Chin poking toward the ceiling, straining the neck
- Losing the scoop so that the spine lifts off the mat
- Not keeping the wrists long and strong

INFORMATION

NUMBER OF REPETITIONS
100 pumps, 10 breaths.

CAUTIONS For neck and back problems, follow the beginner's exercise on page 87; use the modified version, if necessary. For shoulder problems, do not pump the arms.

VISUALIZATION Bounce a ball under your hands.

PRECISION POINTS
- Keep chin into the chest; don't allow the eyes to drift away from the navel.
- Keep the back of the ribs in contact with the mat.
- The shoulder blades stay down the back, as you reach long through the fingers.
- The spine stays softly imprinted on the mat.
- The legs are zipped up in the Pilates stance.

Roll Up

GOALS: ✓ Brings flexibility to the spine, hamstrings and structures along the posterior aspect of the body

✓ Strengthens the abdominal muscles

✓ Trains the spine to move in individual segments rather than in a block

1 **Lie on the mat with your legs lengthened in the Pilates stance, zipped up into a strong centerline, with your feet flexed.** Reach your hands toward the ceiling, directly over the shoulders, with the arms in your shoulder joints and

your ribs funnelled in. When you are ready you will feel lengthened on the mat, with the crown of your head reaching behind you and your heels reaching in the opposite direction; but the backs of your shoulder blades are in contact with the mat, as your hands point to the ceiling.

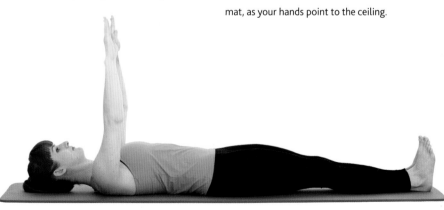

2 **Inhale and bring your chin to your chest.** As you start to roll up, funnel your ribs further and pull your abdominals in deeper to your spine. Peel up off the mat, bone by bone.

3 **Exhale, reaching your hands forward as your powerhouse pulls in, up and back, to create the shape in your spine of a large capital C.** You should feel a strong sense of opposition, as your arms reach forward and your powerhouse lifts up and back.

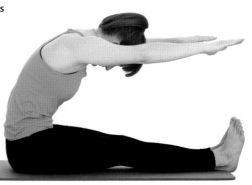

4 **Inhale, scoop your powerhouse and start rolling back, with your tailbone tucking under.** Exhale as you control your journey onto the mat, replacing your spine vertebra by vertebra, until you are lying flat with your shoulders on the mat and your hands toward the ceiling. Begin again immediately and roll up, keeping the movement flowing smoothly.

TRANSITION
Lie in the center of your mat ready for One-Leg Circles.

MODIFICATIONS

For a tight, stiff lower back, keep your knees bent as you roll down and back up; as you reach your arms long, lengthen your legs, then bend them again to roll back.

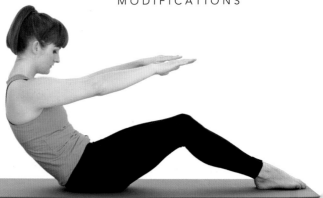

COMMON ERRORS

- Losing the connection of the ribs and the powerhouse, so that the abdominals bulge and the spine arches

- Coming off the mat and lowering onto it with your spine in one block, rather than bone by bone

- The legs lifting as you roll up or down
- The shoulders lifting to the ears

INFORMATION

NUMBER OF REPETITIONS 3–5.

CAUTIONS For a stiff lower back, follow the Modifications. For lower back pain and disc problems, proceed with caution. Refer to the beginner's version Roll Down on page 90 and find the right level for you. It may be necessary to use the beginner's modification or omit the exercise completely. For weak abdominals, do Roll Down on page 90.

VISUALIZATION Your legs are cemented into the mat.

PRECISION POINTS

- Zip the legs up in the center from heel to seat.
- The legs reach away from you as you roll up and down, helping to keep them firmly on the mat.
- A sense of opposition is created, as you reach your hands forward and your waist lifts up and back.
- The ribs and abdominals are kept engaged throughout the move.
- The arms are kept in the shoulder joints, to stop the shoulders lifting toward the ears.

One-Leg Circles

GOALS:
- ✓ Maintains alignment at the hip, knee, pelvis and spine while moving the leg
- ✓ Provides a greater challenge to stability than the beginner's version
- ✓ Engages the buttock muscles and inner thigh
- ✓ Teaches awareness of the centerline

1 **Lie on the mat, draw your right knee in to your chest, then lengthen the leg to the ceiling, with a slight turn-out, into the Pilates stance.** Your left leg should reach long onto the mat, strong into your centerline. Open the front of your chest and use your powerhouse to imprint your spine softly into the mat; you are ready to proceed when you have done this, so that there is no shift when you start to move. The back of your shoulders should be in contact with the mat, with your collar bones softened and your chest open.

2 **Inhale and move your right leg across your body toward the opposite shoulder, reaching long.** Do not allow your right hip to lift off the mat; anchor yourself through your hips, left leg and powerhouse.

3 **Take the leg down along the centerline** to the lowest point in one continuous motion.

Exhale and bring the leg out in line
with the right shoulder, then sweep
it back up to your starting position. There
are three points: across, down and back up.
"Round" the corners, to make a smooth
oval shape in the air with your foot. After

five repetitions, reverse the movement:
out to the side, down and back up. Bring
your right knee in to the chest, then slide it
along the mat. Change legs, and repeat
with the left leg.

TRANSITION Bend your knees and place your feet
on the floor. Lift your arms to the ceiling, then bring
your chin to your chest. Roll up to a sitting position,
articulating your spine as you come up. Bring
yourself forward on the mat for Rolling Like a Ball.

MODIFICATIONS

If your hamstrings limit you, bend the
left leg while circling the right, or refer
to the beginner's version on page 94.
If your neck and/or shoulders are tight,
place your head on a block.

COMMON ERRORS

- Chin poking to the ceiling, which strains the neck
- The lengthened leg bending at the knee

- Losing the scoop of the powerhouse so that the spine lifts off the mat
- Tucking the tail under
- The pelvis "rocking and rolling"

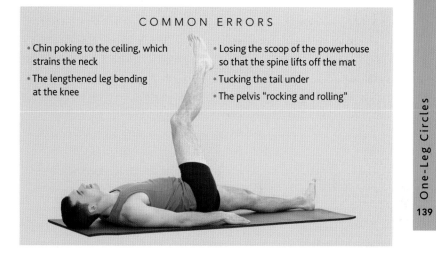

One-Leg Circles

139

INFORMATION

NUMBER OF REPETITIONS

5 each way on each leg.

CAUTIONS For back problems, refer to the beginner's exercise on page 94. If your hip clicks, turn your leg out slightly and engage your backside muscles; make your leg circles smaller.

VISUALIZATION Draw circles with your leg in the sky.

PRECISION POINTS

- The back of the neck is kept lengthened.
- The front of the chest stays softened and open.
- The lengthened leg reaches toward the ceiling through the heel; the leg on the mat reaches away in opposition.
- Maintain the imprint of the spine from the tip of your tailbone to the base of your neck as your leg circles.

Rolling Like a Ball

GOALS: ✓ Trains the powerhouse

✓ Massages the spine

✓ Helps develop control and balance

✓ Works the abdominals and lengthens out the back muscles

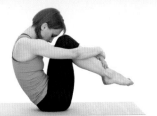

1 **Balance on your sit-bones near the end of the mat, hands holding your ankles, knees slightly apart, with your feet in a Pilates point.** Use the powerhouse to lift your spine and bring your head to your knees. This is your starting position; you should feel very active, in a tight ball shape, with your heels connected to your backside, and your head aiming to be close to your knees. You are held in the balance by your abdominals—not by your shoulders elevating.

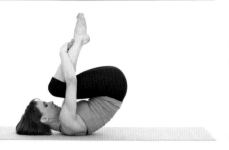

2 **Inhale and roll back, initiating the move from your abdominals.** Maintain the ball shape with a C-curve, and pull firmly into the centerline.

3 **Roll to the base of your shoulders, not onto your head and neck.** Exhale and roll up, using your abdominals, not your biceps.

TRANSITION Move to the center of the mat, balance on your sit-bones, then draw your right knee in, with left hand on right knee, and right hand on right ankle. Lengthen your left leg away. Tuck the tailbone under and roll back for the Single Leg Stretch.

MODIFICATIONS

For knee problems, refer to the beginner's version with the hands behind the thighs, on page 98.

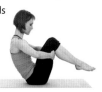

COMMON ERRORS

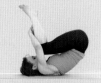

- Not using the powerhouse to make a C-curve in the spine and rolling on a flat back
- Initiating the roll-back by tipping the head back
- Throwing the feet forward as you come back up
- Pulling on the arms to roll back up

INFORMATION

NUMBER OF REPETITIONS 6–8.

CAUTIONS For osteoporosis, omit any rolling exercises if you have bone-density problems more severe than osteopenia. If you have a significant scoliosis, omit this exercise. For back problems, proceed with caution; if you have disc problems, omit this exercise. If you have knee problems, hold behind the thigh.

VISUALIZATION Roll the spine like a wheel.

PRECISION POINTS
- Keep your shape!
- The abdominals, not the biceps, work to pull you up.
- Roll to the tip of the shoulder blades.
- The abdominals keep the lower back lifted out of the pelvis.
- The shoulder blades slide down the back.

Abdominal Five Series: Single Leg Stretch

GOALS: ✓ Trains strength and endurance in the abdominals

✓ Promotes alignment

✓ Brings stabilization of the trunk, as the limbs move rhythmically

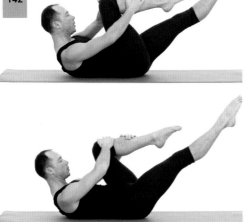

TRANSITION Bring your knees in to your chest and hold your ankles, ready for the Double Leg Stretch. Keep your chin to your chest.

1 Lie in the center of your mat with your chin to your chest, right leg pulled in and left leg lengthened at a 45° angle. Your right knee is in line with your right shoulder, right hand on the ankle and left hand on the right knee.

2 Inhale and change legs; draw your left leg in firmly in line with your left shoulder, and lengthen your right leg out to a 45° angle. Keep anchored strongly to the mat. Then exhale and switch legs again. Stretch the lengthened leg from the hip along your centerline, so that your heels reach the same point in space.

MODIFICATIONS

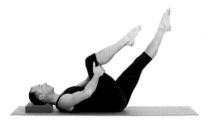

For knee problems, place your hands behind your thigh rather than on the knee joint. **If you have difficulties with your neck,** or if it fatigues, use a block under your head. **If you have a weak or vulnerable back,** refer to the beginner's version on page 102.

COMMON ERRORS

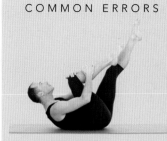

- The trunk rotating as the legs move
- Losing the midline, with the legs wandering out to the side, away from the centerline
- The powerhouse losing the scoop as the legs change
- Losing the connection of the shoulders down the back
- The tailbone tucking under

INFORMATION

NUMBER OF REPETITIONS 6–10.

CAUTIONS For knee, neck and back issues, refer to the Modifications.

VISUALIZATION Find an imagery point in space along your centerline, and aim each heel to that spot.

PRECISION POINTS

- The powerhouse is active in imprinting the spine and maintaining your box throughout.
- The legs glide along the centerline.
- The shoulders stay off the mat, but away from the ears.
- The eyes are kept on the navel, and the chin to the chest.

Abdominal Five Series: Double Leg Stretch

GOALS:
✓ Trains strength and stamina of the abdominals
✓ Teaches opposition in two directions from a strong center
✓ Trains a full exhalation, to gain a full inhalation to coordinate with the movement

1 **Lie on your back with your chin and your knees to your chest, knees slightly apart.** Place hands on ankles; your spine should be firmly imprinted into the mat from the tailbone to the tips of your shoulder blades.

2 **Inhale and lengthen your limbs out, with your arms by your ears and your legs at a 45° angle in Pilates stance.** Your head should stay lifted without movement; your abdominals should draw deeply in to the spine, with your back ribs staying imprinted into the mat.

3 **Exhale and sweep your arms round to your sides,** pull your knees in from the abdominals, and hold your ankles as you hug your legs back into the starting position.

MODIFICATIONS

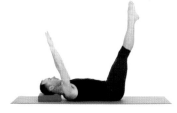

If you struggle to keep your head up, use a block underneath it, and bring your legs more toward the ceiling.

If your abdominals are not strong enough initially, take your legs toward the ceiling, as in the beginner's version on page 104; as you get stronger you will be able to progressively lower your legs.

COMMON ERRORS

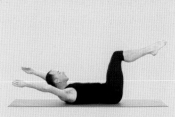

- The head dropping back
- Losing the imprint of the spine, with the abdominals lifting
- The tailbone coming off the mat in the hug position
- The shoulders lifting to the ears, and the ribs popping toward the ceiling

INFORMATION

NUMBER OF REPETITIONS 6–10.

CAUTIONS For knee pain, avoid pressure through the knee joints, and place the hands behind the thighs. For shoulder problems, keep the movement of the arms small. For back and neck problems, proceed with caution and refer to the beginner's version on page 104.

VISUALIZATION Stretch out long, pull in strong.

PRECISION POINTS
- Keep the tip of the tail on the mat to avoid tucking the pelvis under.
- The legs are strongly wrapped into the centerline.
- The spine and the back of the ribs stay imprinted on the mat as the limbs lengthen away.

Abdominal Five Series: Single Straight-Leg Stretch "Scissors"

GOALS: ✓ Trains the abdominals to maintain stability of the trunk while the legs move dynamically

✓ Challenges the strength and stamina of the powerhouse

✓ Brings flexibility to the hamstrings, with stability of the torso

1 Lie on your back and lengthen your legs toward the ceiling, with your hands on the right ankle; your head should be up, with your eyes on your navel. Your spine is imprinted on the mat, from the tailbone to the tips of your shoulder blades; don't let the tail tuck under. Find the rib/shoulder-blade connection, with your elbows wide. Simultaneously pull the right leg toward you with a double pulse as the other leg reaches away along the midline, in a scissor-like movement.

2 Switch the legs in a fluid motion, taking hold of the left ankle for a double pulse. Your abdominals should be pulled in deeply, to keep the torso stable. The exercise keeps moving with a strong and dynamic pulse-pulse rhythm as the leg comes in. Inhale for one repetition (both legs scissored); exhale for the next.

TRANSITION Take both legs toward the ceiling and lower the head, to get ready for the Double Straight-Leg Stretch

MODIFICATIONS

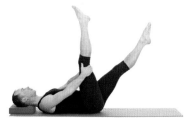

For a weak neck, use a block under the head. **To accommodate difficulties with flexibility,** particularly in the hamstrings, place your hands on your leg in a position where it is still possible to keep your tailbone and spine on the mat. Reduce the range of movement of your legs.

COMMON ERRORS

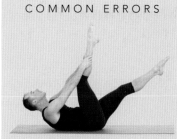

- Rolling up the top half of the body
- Not keeping the legs lengthened, but letting them bend
- Losing the imprint of the spine, so that the trunk bobs around on the mat during the exercise

INFORMATION

NUMBER OF REPETITIONS 6–10.

CAUTIONS If your neck tires, rest it intermittently.

VISUALIZATION Move the legs like a pair of scissors.

PRECISION POINTS
- One leg lowers to the point where the other leg has come in, so that they are equidistant apart when scissored.

- The tips of the shoulder blades are kept on the mat, and only the top of the shoulders lifts.
- The trunk stays square, with no rotation as the legs move.
- The movement is initiated from the powerhouse.

Abdominal Five Series: Double Straight-Leg Stretch "Lower Lifts'

GOALS: ✓ Strengthens and builds stamina in the abdominals

✓ Develops control, maintaining the work in the abdominals while lowering the legs

1 **Lie on your back with your legs up in the Pilates stance, perpendicular to the mat.** Lift your head using your abdominals, and place your hands behind your head; do not interlink your fingers— one hand should be placed on top of the other. Your eyes should be on your navel, with your elbows in the periphery of your vision. Your abdominals should be deeply engaged, with a strong sense of the ribs being pulled in. The tips of your shoulder blades should still touch the mat, but your shoulders should be away from your ears. Your backside and inner thighs should be active; this will help take the tension off the front of your thighs.

2 Inhale and deepen the powerhouse, and then, with control, reach your legs away to lower them, for a count of 3. Exhale, using your abdominals to return your legs to the perpendicular for a count of 1, keeping your sacrum on the mat.

TRANSITION Bring both knees in to your chest to prepare for Criss-Cross.

For tight hamstrings, a tight lower back or weak abdominals, use one of the following two Modifications:

1 Make a diamond with your hands and place then under your sacrum, with your head up; keep the range of motion of your legs smaller.

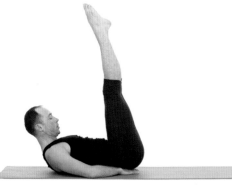

2 Bend your knees to a tabletop position, with your head up and your hands behind your head; keep the movement of the legs small.

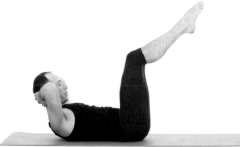

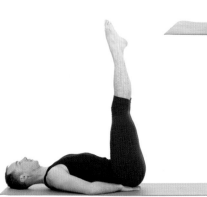

For a weak neck, make a diamond with your hands and place them under your sacrum, with your head on the mat. Keep the movement of the legs small, to maintain the imprint of your spine on the mat.

COMMON ERRORS

- The back lifting off the mat—if this begins to happen, you have lowered the legs too far
- The abdominals losing the scoop so that the abdomen pops up to the ceiling

- Rolling the tip of the tailbone off the mat as the legs return to the starting position

INFORMATION

NUMBER OF REPETITIONS 6–10.

CAUTIONS This exercise requires both strength and control, with the abdominals taking the load of both legs as they lower, so if your abdominals are not strong enough to keep your spine on the mat as the legs lower, use the Modifications or omit this exercise until you are stronger. For back issues and injuries, omit the exercise. For neck issues, leave the head down on the mat and follow the Modifications.

VISUALIZATION Resist a spring in order to lower the legs; control the recoil of the spring to lift the legs.

PRECISION POINTS
- The spine *must* be maintained in contact with the mat for the duration of the move, using the scoop.
- The tailbone does not lift as the legs return to the upright position.
- The elbows are kept wide, the shoulders down and the ribs in.
- Use the wrap in the legs to support the powerhouse; the legs are pressed into the centerline.

Abdominal Five Series: Criss-Cross

GOALS: ✓ Builds strength and stamina of the abdominals

✓ Specifically works the oblique abdominal muscles

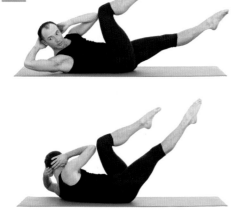

1 **Lie on your back, with your knees pulled into the chest and your hands behind your head, overlapped but not intertwined.** Inhale and draw your right knee in, in line with your right shoulder. Lift your upper body and reach your left elbow to the right knee; touch it if you can. Your right elbow should reach behind you, without touching the floor; your eyes should follow the right elbow.

2 **Exhale and keep the lift from your ribs,** so that your shoulders remain lifted off the mat and you can criss-cross to bring your right elbow to your left knee, with your eyes on the left elbow as it reaches back.

TRANSITION Bring both knees in to your chest in the center; hold the back of your thighs and come to a seated position for the Spine Stretch Forward.

MODIFICATIONS

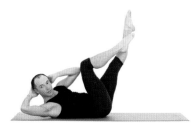

For weaker backs or abdominals, take the lengthened leg toward the ceiling.

COMMON ERRORS

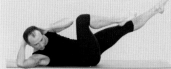

- Rocking and rolling around on the mat, rather than working from the lift of the abdominals
- The shoulders sliding up to the ears, the elbows coming in, and the hands pulling on the neck
- Losing the height of the upper body during the criss-cross from side to side

INFORMATION

NUMBER OF REPETITIONS 6–10.

CAUTIONS For neck issues, omit the exercise, as there is no modification for weak necks. For recent back injuries or ongoing back issues, care is needed, due to the rotation of the spine; it may be necessary to omit this exercise.

VISUALIZATION Wring the ribs out to lift and twist them.

PRECISION POINTS

- Avoid rushing this exercise to finish it quickly, or you will miss some of the benefits of it!
- The lift is maintained throughout from the upper abdominals.
- The hips and lower spine are kept anchored on the mat.
- The box is held, and the legs stay strong into the centerline—don't let them fall out of the frame.
- Both heels reach to the same point in space.

Spine Stretch Forward

GOALS:
- ✓ Brings flexibility to the spine and hamstrings
- ✓ Teaches how to sit tall and lift out of the hips
- ✓ Promotes articulation of the spine

1 **Sit tall on the mat, growing long through the crown of your head as if you are sitting against a wall.** Place your legs straight out, just wider than shoulder-width, with your feet flexed and knees facing the ceiling. Hold your arms parallel to the floor and shoulder-width apart. Inhale and grow taller, lifting out of the hips and engaging your bottom muscles. Every time you come into a sitting position in Pilates you should have a sense of being active from the very base: the pelvic floor is lifted, the seat muscles work to give you a little "perch," your scoop is active and you feel as if you have grown taller. You are now ready to continue this exercise.

2 **Exhale and roll down, bringing your chin to your chest and lifting your abdominals; round yourself up and over.** Create opposition in a deep stretch, with your spine lifted into a C-curve and your navel pulling back, while the energy from your arms reaches forward; lengthen through your heels to the opposite wall. Exhale completely. Then inhale and initiate rolling the spine back up from the lowest vertebra, stacking bone on bone so that you are sitting tall, with the crown of the head reaching to the ceiling.

TRANSITION Bend your knees, draw your heels into your seat and hold your ankles, ready for the Open-Leg Rocker—Preparation.

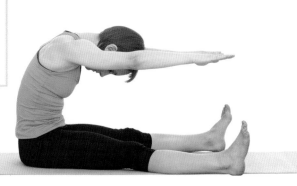

MODIFICATIONS

For tight hamstrings or a tight lower back, sit on a block so that your shoulders are directly over your hips; or softly bend your knees (see the beginner's version on page 108 or the Modifications).

If you have fragile or painful shoulders, slide your hands forward along the mat between your legs.

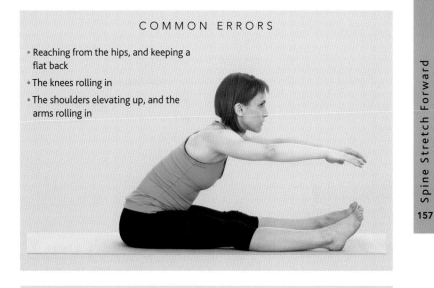

COMMON ERRORS

- Reaching from the hips, and keeping a flat back
- The knees rolling in
- The shoulders elevating up, and the arms rolling in

INFORMATION

NUMBER OF REPETITIONS 5.

CAUTIONS If you have a stiff lower back or back and shoulder problems, follow the Modifications above or the beginner's Modifications on page 108.

VISUALIZATION Squeeze a beach ball between your thighs to create the lift, then round yourself over the ball.

PRECISION POINTS

- Keep the feet flexed.
- Keep the knees facing the ceiling.
- Use the powerhouse to make a lifted arc in the spine.
- Do not flop forward from the hips.
- Ensure that you roll the spine up as if you were rolling up against a wall, not in one block.
- Maintain an active backside, to keep you lifted throughout the move.

Open-Leg Rocker—Preparation

GOALS: ✓ Challenges control, balance and coordination

✓ Brings flexibility to the spine and hamstrings

1 **Sit on the mat with your knees bent, and draw your heels in toward you.** Hold the outside of your ankles and, using your abdominals, lift your feet off the mat and tip backward to balance on your tailbone. Your knees should be shoulder-width apart, your feet softly pointed, and your shoulders down the back. You are in an active balance, held in that little "point" by a deep scoop, to lift the spine and prevent you tipping forward or back. Your shoulder blades must not elevate in an effort to help keep you there.

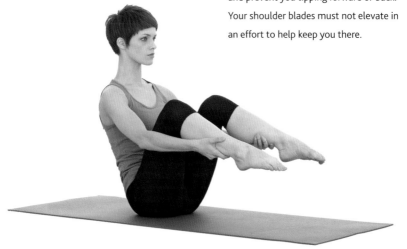

2 **Breathing naturally, lengthen your right leg, keeping your chest and powerhouse lifted.** Bend, then switch legs, maintaining your balance.

3 **Lengthen your right leg again, then bring your left leg up to join it.** The back of your neck should remain long, with the chest lifted.

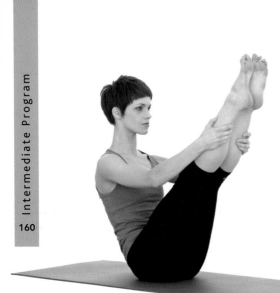

4 **Keeping everything else the same, close your legs; then open them again to shoulder width apart.** Close them again, so that the legs are zipped up in the centerline.

> **TRANSITION** Keep your legs reaching long, release the ankles and roll your upper body down to the mat, with the legs at a 90° angle, ready for Corkscrew I. Alternatively, bend your knees and roll your upper body down, ready for Corkscrew I.

MODIFICATIONS

For tight hamstrings and general flexibility issues, adjust your hand position; aim to come as few places as possible away from the ankles, so that you are working toward the ideal of the exercise. For very tight hamstrings, hold behind the thigh and bend the knees, so that your lower legs are parallel to the floor—and just balance there. To build up to the full balance, start with one toe on the mat, taking one leg at a time long.

COMMON ERRORS

- The shoulders rising and sliding around the chest wall

- Keeping the balance by holding onto the legs with the arms, rather than using the lift in the powerhouse

- Losing the frame so that the legs fall out to the sides

INFORMATION

NUMBER OF REPETITIONS

1 repetition of the whole sequence, with a brief hold in the full balance.

CAUTIONS If you have a tender tailbone, it may be too uncomfortable to proceed. For recent back injuries or disc problems, omit the exercise. For a weak lower back, weak abdominals or tight hamstrings, follow the Modifications.

VISUALIZATION In the full balance, lift your chest to the sun and feel the warmth.

PRECISION POINTS

- The chest stays lifted, with the eyes on the horizon.
- The box is kept square.
- The powerhouse keeps the abdomen lifted out of the pelvis.

Corkscrew I

GOALS:
✓ Develops stability in the trunk

✓ Strengthens the legs and lower abdominals

✓ Enables movement of the legs separately from the pelvis

1 **Lie on your back, with your arms by your sides and your collar bones open and soft.** Your legs should be directly toward the ceiling, zipped up strongly together in the Pilates stance. Your powerhouse will firmly imprint your spine on the mat, from your tailbone to the top of the head, so that there is no shift in your torso during the exercise. The backs of your shoulders are also in contact with the mat, and not rolled forward.

2 **Inhale and take your legs as one across to the left,** in line with your shoulders; your right hip should stay firmly glued to the mat.

3 **Circle your legs down and to the center,** ensuring that your spine stays on the mat.

4 **Exhale and, scooping your powerhouse deeply, circle your legs round to the right, then up and then back to the center.** Inhale to reverse the circle.

> **TRANSITION** In the center, bring your knees into your chest, with chin to chest and hands behind your thighs, and roll up to a sitting position for Saw.

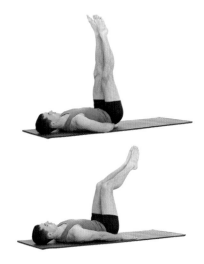

MODIFICATIONS

For tight hamstrings or a weak back, use one of the following Modifications that best suits your needs:

1 Make a diamond with your hands and place them under your sacrum; keep the circles of the legs small.

2 Soften your knees to allow you to keep your sacrum on the mat and your spine imprinted, as you make small circles.

COMMON ERRORS

- Losing the imprint of the spine on the mat so that the lower back lifts and the chin pokes up
- The legs not moving as one, with one heel moving forward relative to the other
- The shoulders rolling forward, with the hands gripping the mat

INFORMATION

NUMBER OF REPETITIONS

2–4 in each direction.

CAUTIONS For recent back injury, omit the exercise. For a weak back and abdominals, follow the Modifications.

VISUALIZATION Your feet trace the outline of a circle on the ceiling.

PRECISION POINTS

- The chest remains open with the arms soft on the mat.
- The hips stay on the mat throughout the circle.
- Every bone of the spine is in contact with the mat, and the neck lengthens through the crown of the head.
- The upper abdominal muscles work to keep the ribs in.
- The legs remain zipped up together.

Saw

GOALS: ✓ Works the spine's range of motion into rotation, with the powerhouse decompressing the spine

✓ Trains the abdominals in a sitting position

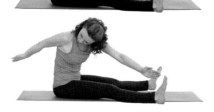

1 **Sit on the mat, with your feet just wider than the mat, your legs long and feet flexed.** Grow tall out of your hips. Your arms should be long out to the sides, but still within your vision. Your powerhouse, pelvic floor and seat muscles should feel as if they are lifting you to sit tall, but your pelvis and legs should feel as if they have roots into the mat; you are active and strong.

2 **Inhale as you engage your abdominals to lift and lengthen the spine,** twisting from the waist to the right.

3 **Exhale and reach your left little finger past your right little toe; reach your right hand back and up.** Deepen the opposition, sawing your little finger past your toe for a count of 1, 2; then reach even further for 3, until you have no more air left in your lungs. Inhale and use your abdominals to lift the spine, twisting to the left to repeat the action on that side.

TRANSITION Bring your arms and legs together, then roll down onto your front for Swan Neck Roll.

MODIFICATIONS

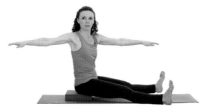

For a stiff lower back or tight hamstrings, sit on a block to bring your shoulders over your pelvis. **For shoulder and back issues**, refer to the Modifications of the beginner's exercise on page 112.

COMMON ERRORS

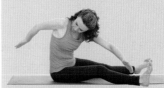

• The knees rolling and bending
• Rotating from the shoulders, rather than lifting and twisting from the waist and ribs
• Lifting the opposite hip as you reach past the little toe
• Losing the C-curve with the full reach

INFORMATION

NUMBER OF REPETITIONS 3–5.

....

CAUTIONS For shoulder problems, either follow the Modifications to the beginner's exercise on page 112 or omit this exercise. For back problems, exercise care with the combination of twist and bend; or follow the Modifications to the beginner's exercise on page 112 or omit this exercise.

....

VISUALIZATION Open the lid of a jar as you twist.

PRECISION POINTS
• The pelvis is set in cement on the mat, so that it does not lift as you reach and the heels stay level.
• The knees stay facing the ceiling, with the energy of the legs reaching through the heels.
• Find a deep C-curve as you reach your hands away.
• With the inhale, use the powerhouse to lift you taller as you twist.
• The eyes track the hand that reaches back, with the palm to the ceiling.

Swan Neck Roll

1 **Lie on the mat; press your legs together in the Pilates stance, with your hands under your shoulders, and your elbows lifted and held firmly in to your sides.** Your powerhouse should be lifted into your spine, and your shoulders should slide down your back.

When you are set up for this exercise, you feel very long and active as you lie on your front; to scoop your abdominals, imagine there is an ice cube on the mat! As you scoop, your spine will lengthen, rather than create a "hollow" in the lower back; the back of your neck should be long, so keep your chin gently tucked in.

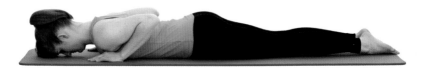

2 **Inhale and initiate a lengthening of your spine off the mat, by rolling your nose along the mat; lift your chest, creating a long spine.** Use your abdominals to create the lift, rather than pushing up through your hands. Your pelvis should stay on the mat.

3 **Breathe naturally** and rotate your head to the left.

4 Take your chin to your chest.

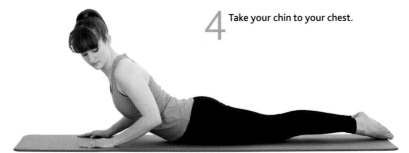

5 **Roll your chin round to your center.**

6 **Continue to roll your chin around to the right, then return your head to the center.** Keep your shoulders sliding down your back. Pull in your abdominals and grow longer through the crown of your head, to lengthen back down to the mat.

TRANSITION Sit up on the mat from the rest position, then roll back down on to the mat in preparation for the Shoulder Bridge position.

REST POSITION

Tuck your tailbone under and lift your abdominals to create a C-curve, so your stomach and ribs are lifted off your thighs, with your knees slightly apart. Inhale to fill your lungs to their full capacity; on the exhale, use your powerhouse to deepen the stretch of your lower back. Take care if you have hip and knee problems; for tight shoulders, bring your arms by your side.

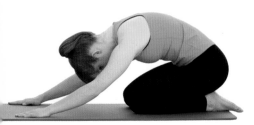

MODIFICATIONS

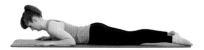

For a stiff lower back or other back issues, keep your feet hip-width apart and lift only part of the way. **For wrist, elbow and shoulder problems**, slide your hands slightly further forward, keep your forearms on the mat and lift only part of the way.

COMMON ERRORS

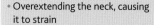

- Overextending the neck, causing it to strain
- Sinking in the shoulders and lower back
- Pushing up through the hands, not from the powerhouse
- Belly extending onto the mat

INFORMATION

NUMBER OF REPETITIONS 1–2 with the neck roll, 1 lift to the center.

CAUTIONS For wrist, elbow, shoulder and back issues, follow the Modifications. Ensure a strong powerhouse throughout the move; the lower back should not pinch.

VISUALIZATION Imagine your neck growing as long as a swan's.

PRECISION POINTS
- Lengthening is through the abdominals, to lift the body.
- The ribs are kept in; this will help keep you lifted.
- The focus for the eyes is toward the horizon.
- The neck is long, and the shoulders are down the back.

Shoulder Bridge Preparation

GOALS: ✓ Articulates the spine

✓ Controls and stabilizes the pelvis and lower trunk

✓ Strengthens the hamstrings and buttocks

✓ Opens up the front of the hips

1 **Lie on your back with your knees bent, feet flat and legs parallel, in line with the hips.** Your collar bones should be open and soft, with your palms pressing into the mat and the back of your neck lengthened.

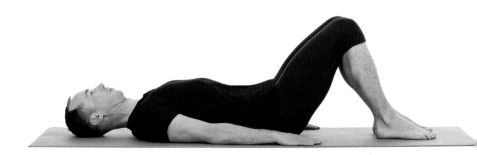

2 **Inhale and press your pelvis to the ceiling in one line.** Reach through your knees to open up your hips, while your tailbone reaches to the back of your calves.

3 **Exhale and roll your spine down, from the chest first, placing each vertebra onto the mat one by one.** Create a sense of length by keeping the back of your neck long and your tailbone reaching to the back of your legs for the whole of the roll-down. Repeat 3–5 times.

4 **As a progression, you can add in leg lifts.**
Set up as in steps 1 and 2, but press your legs together in the centerline. Lift your right leg level with the left leg and lengthen it. Keep your hips level and your weight evenly distributed.

5 **Inhale and kick the leg up to the ceiling, with your foot soft and your hands pressing into the mat.** Your shoulders should remain open and your neck long. Exhale and lengthen the leg, parallel to the weight-bearing leg. Kick the same leg three times, then replace the foot and change legs.

TRANSITION
Lengthen your legs on the mat, then roll onto your side in a straight line along the back edge of the mat, for the Side Kick series.

MODIFICATIONS

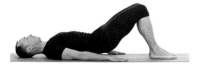

Keep the range of movement smaller. Practise the Fundamentals Clock (see page 69) to work toward the bigger Bridge movement.

COMMON ERRORS

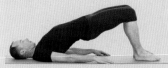

- The ribs and the abdomen flaring to the ceiling, due to the powerhouse switching off
- Pressing down through the head, neck and arms to get the lift of the pelvis—this will strain the neck
- Wobbling when lifting and lowering the pelvis, losing the box
- The pelvis dipping when lifting a leg

INFORMATION

NUMBER OF REPETITIONS 3–5 lifts of the pelvis; 3 lifts on each leg if doing the progression.

CAUTIONS For neck, back or knee issues, follow the Modifications.

VISUALIZATION Place one vertebra at a time onto the mat, like the links in a bicycle chain.

PRECISION POINTS
- The collarbone stays soft and open, and the neck is lengthened.
- Keep a strong centerline and maintain the box.
- The ribs stay flush with your front, with the powerhouse active.
- The hips stay level when lifting the leg.

Side Kick Series: Front/Back

GOALS: ✓ Tones, lengthens and strengthens the legs, hips and abdominals

✓ Provides a dynamic stretch to the hamstrings

✓ Helps develop stability and balance

1 **Lying on your side, line yourself along the back edge of the mat.** Come up onto your elbow, with your head on your hand and your neck long. Rest your top hand on the floor in front of you, with your elbow pressed into your hip. Use your abdominals to lift your waist, so that you are in a long, lean line. At this point your powerhouse is so active that you should feel the energy reaching through the top of your head, while your legs reach away strongly in the opposite direction.

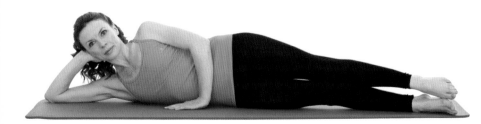

2 Breathe naturally, lift both legs together in the Pilates stance, then bring your legs forward and lower, so that your feet are at the front corner of the mat, or at a 45° angle. The slight bend in the hips will make you feel more stable.

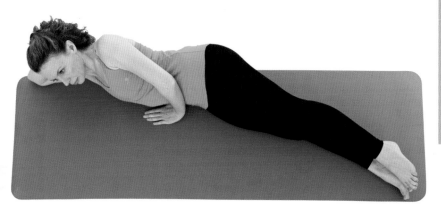

3 Breathe naturally, lift your top leg to hip height; kick forward with a double pulse: kick-kick. Keep your hips and shoulders stacked, and your top leg parallel with the floor.

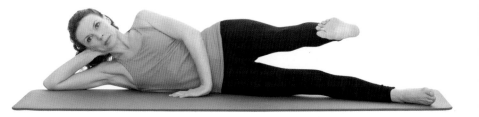

4 **Kick your leg back long and strong from the hip;** keep your backside muscles firm, to take your leg behind you.

TRANSITION Bring your top heel in line with your bottom heel, with a slight turn-out, ready for Up/Down.

MODIFICATIONS

For neck or shoulder problems, use a block under your head, with your bottom arm lengthened forward on the mat. Find a block of the correct height so that your neck is in line with the rest of your spine. It is important to treat both sides of the body same, even if the problem is only one-sided. **For hip problems and hip replacements,** your movements should stay small and controlled.

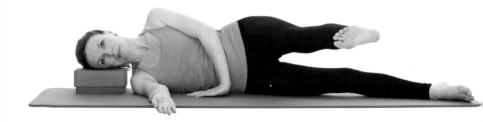

COMMON ERRORS

- The top leg swinging around without control
- Hips and shoulders rocking and rolling!

- Losing the long line of the spine, causing it to bend and extend with the movement of the leg

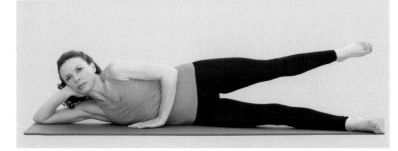

INFORMATION

NUMBER OF REPETITIONS 5–10.

CAUTIONS Keep the range of movement smaller for hip problems and hip replacements. If you are unable to rest your head on your hand, due to neck or shoulder problems, follow the Modifications.

VISUALIZATION Draw a semicircle with your foot, parallel to the floor.

PRECISION POINTS
- Keep the gaze forward.
- Keep the box.
- The top leg stays level with the hip and reaches long out of it.

Side Kick Series: Up/Down

GOALS: ✓ Tones, lengthens and strengthens the legs, hips and abdominals

✓ Works the flexibility of the inner thigh

✓ Helps train stability and balance

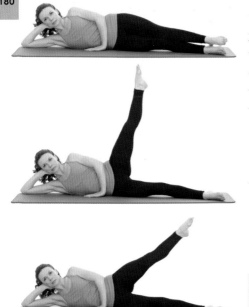

1 **Lie on your side at the back edge of the mat, with your head on your bottom hand, your top hand on the mat and your feet at the front corner.** Your top leg should be in line with your bottom leg, heel-to-heel, with the top leg slightly turned out.

2 **Inhale and, keeping your hips stacked,** lift the top leg toward the ceiling.

3 **Exhale as you reach the leg long to lower it.**

TRANSITION Return to the starting position for Passé.

MODIFICATIONS

If you have neck and shoulder problems that restrict you placing your head on your hand, use a block under your head, so that your neck does not feel any strain. **For hip problems,** including hip replace - ments, be mindful and use a smaller range of movement.

COMMON ERRORS

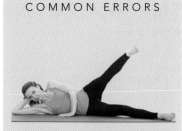

- The top hip falling back as the leg lifts
- The top leg becoming "soggy"
- Waist collapsing to the floor
- Losing the shoulder connection

INFORMATION

NUMBER OF REPETITIONS 5.

CAUTIONS For hip problems, includ- ing hip replacements and hips that "clunk," keep the movement smaller and work with active seat muscles. Follow the Modifications if you are unable to support your head on your hand, due to neck or shoulder problems.

VISUALIZATION Kick the leg up straight and long, then bring it down straight and strong.

PRECISION POINTS
- The hips stay stacked.
- The eyes focus on a point in front, so that the neck is lengthened.
- As the leg lifts, the trunk stays square, with the powerhouse active.

Side Kick Series: Passé

GOALS: ✓ Challenges balance

✓ Tones, lengthens and strengthens the abdominals, buttocks and thighs

✓ Brings flexibility to the hips, and stability of the pelvis

1 In your side-lying position, align your top leg on your lower leg, heel-to-heel, so that there is a slight turn-out of the top leg. Slide your big toe along the inside of your bottom leg.

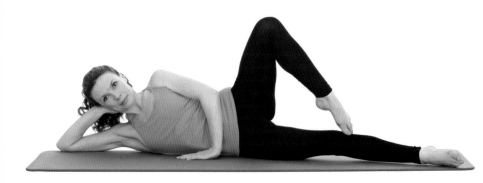

2 **Take your top knee to your ear,** with your hips open and stacked, and breathe naturally.

3 **Straighten your leg,** reaching to get it behind your ear and maintaining the alignment in your hips.

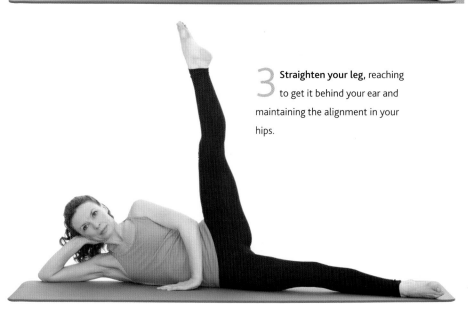

4 **Lower the leg, reaching it long.**
Repeat 3 times, then reverse the move for another three repetitions: kick the leg up long behind the ear, bend, then slide the big toe along the lower leg to straighten the top leg.

TRANSITION Lengthen the top leg over the bottom leg, maintaining it at hip height, ready for Circles.

MODIFICATIONS

For reduced flexibility in the hips or other hip issues, slide the top toes along the inside of the lower leg; do not extend the leg toward the ceiling. **If you have neck or shoulder issues,** use a block under your head, and extend your bottom arm out in front of you. Use a block of the correct height so that it fills the gap between the mat and your head, without straining your neck.

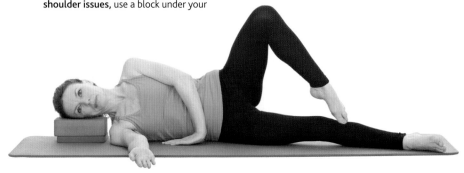

COMMON ERRORS

- The top hip falls back as the leg lifts
- Chest rolling forward
- Bending the spine, with the eyes watching the legs

- Losing the lift of the powerhouse so that the abdominals sink onto the mat

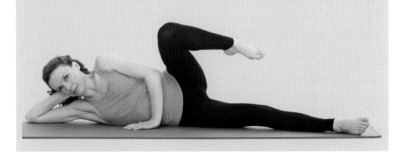

INFORMATION

NUMBER OF REPETITIONS

3 each way, on each leg.

CAUTIONS For hip problems, follow the Modifications, or omit the exercise. For hips that "clunk," ensure you have your wrap engaged; if that doesn't get rid of the clunking, follow the Modi - fications until your hip stability has improved sufficiently to cope with the larger movement.

VISUALIZATION Draw a line on the bottom leg with the big toe.

PRECISION POINTS

- The abdominals stay lifted and off the mat.
- Mark all points of the movement— do not cut corners: bend for 1, lift for 2, lengthen for 3, lower long for 4.
- Keep the spine long from your crown to the tip of your tailbone.

Side Kick Series: Circles

GOALS:
- ✓ Trains balance
- ✓ Tones, lengthens and strengthens the abdominals, buttocks and thighs
- ✓ Brings stability to the pelvis and trunk, while the leg moves in the hip

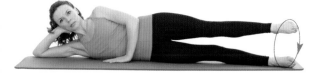

1 **In your side-lying position,** reach your top leg long out of the hip, to lift it to hip height.

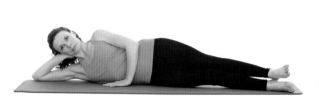

2 **Make small circles with the top leg— the instep of your top foot brushing the heel of your bottom foot.** Repeat 5–8 times, then reverse the circles with the top leg at hip height. Breathe naturally throughout.

TRANSITION Lift the top leg and place the foot on the mat in front of the lower leg; hold your ankle with your top hand, ready for Inner Thigh Lifts and Circles.

MODIFICATIONS

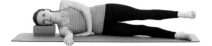

For shoulder and neck problems, use a
block of the right size under your head.

COMMON ERRORS

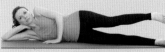

- Letting the ankle go "soggy," so that
  the foot and knee roll in
- Losing the lift of the waist
- Watching the feet, causing the spine
  to flex
- Pelvis moving around as the leg
  moves, when it should remain stable

INFORMATION

NUMBER OF REPETITIONS 5–8.

CAUTIONS For neck and shoulder
problems, follow the Modifications.

VISUALIZATION The instep "kisses"
the heel as it brushes past in tight
circles.

PRECISION POINTS
- The top leg is active and lengthened,
  without the knee being braced.
- The circles come from the hip, not
  the ankle.
- The hips stay stacked one on top of
  the other.
- The neck is long and the eyes forward.

Side Kick Series: Inner Thigh Lifts and Circles

GOALS: ✓ Creates muscle balance in the thighs

✓ Stretches out the hip and buttock of the leg that has just worked

1 **In your side-lying position, bend the top leg and place the foot on the mat.** Hold the ankle with your top hand and work your top knee to the ceiling. Engage your powerhouse and maintain the length in your spine; do not let the spine flex to accommodate bending the top leg and bringing the foot onto the mat. It is quite normal for most people to feel a stretch or an opening of the top hip in this position.

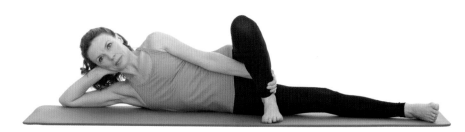

2 **Breathe naturally and lift the lower leg from the hip, with a straight knee.** Lengthen the leg to lower it, reaching long out of the hip; do not let it touch the mat. To challenge the inner thigh more, lift it twice before lowering it.

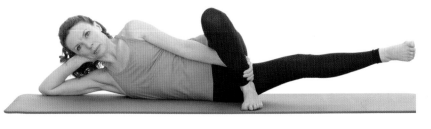

3 **After the last lift,** keep the leg lifted and make large circles forward 5–8 times.

4 **Then reverse the circle** 5–8 times.

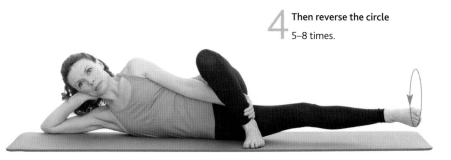

TRANSITION Slide the top leg over the lower leg to set up for Beats on the Belly (see below), as a transition to turning to the other side so that you can work the other leg. After you have worked both sides, bring your legs together, bend both knees and come up to a sitting position for Teaser I Leg.

BEATS ON THE BELLY

1 **Lying on your front, place your forehead on your hands.** Lengthen both legs, pressing the back of your thighs to the ceiling. Beat the heels together for a count of 10, with a snappy tempo.

MODIFICATIONS

For stiff or problematic hips and knees, place your top knee bent on the mat in front of you.

For neck and shoulder problems, use a block of the right height under your head.

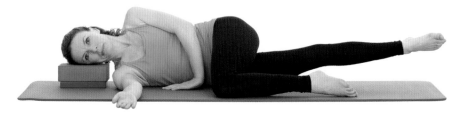

COMMON ERRORS

- Losing the stacking of the hips, and the top hip rolling back
- Working from the foot, not from the hip

- Not maintaining the length in the lower leg, and letting the knee bend

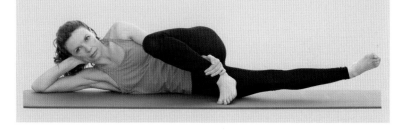

INFORMATION

NUMBER OF REPETITIONS 5–8.

CAUTIONS For tight hips and knees, do not hold the ankle; if necessary, follow the Modifications. For neck issues, follow the Modifications

VISUALIZATION Balance a book on the inside of your knee, and don't let it slide off.

PRECISION POINTS

- The gaze stays forward to maintain a lengthened neck and spine.
- Lengthen the moving leg throughout.
- Keep the toes and knee facing forward, so that you lift from the inner thigh.

Teaser I Leg

GOALS: ✓ Strengthens the powerhouse

✓ Stabilizes the pelvis and lower trunk

✓ Promotes sequential movement of the spine

✓ Prepares for the full Teaser series

1 **Sit on the mat, with your knees bent and legs pressed together, keeping your knees level.** Lengthen the right leg in a slight Pilates stance. Sit back on your sit-bones, with a C-curve in your lower back, chest lifted and fingers reaching to your lifted foot. In the set-up position your scoop should hold you in a point just off your tailbone: you are not sitting upright and you are not slumped backward. Your inner thighs are very active and pressed together.

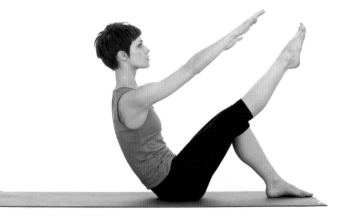

2 **Inhale and initiate a roll of the spine,** by pulling your abdominals in further as your pelvis rolls under; place one vertebra at a time onto the mat, with control.

3 **As you lengthen fully onto the mat,** reach your arms over your head.

4 **Exhale, lift your arms to the ceiling and, following your arms,** lightly roll up off the mat, reversing the move one vertebra at a time.

5 **Float up to a seated position on your sit-bones, with a C-curve in your spine and your chest open and lifted.** Repeat 3–4 times, then scissor your legs to lift your left leg, placing your right foot on the mat, and repeat. When you are able to complete Teaser I Leg keeping your abdominals engaged, challenge yourself further by lifting your arms to your ears and keeping them there for the whole of the move, with your sides lengthened.

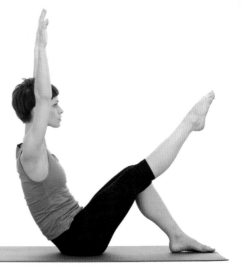

TRANSITION Lift your other leg and balance on your sit-bones, with your fingers reaching toward your toes, when you are ready for Teaser I. If you need to continue to work on Teaser I Leg before progressing to the full Teaser I, then roll down to the mat, lift an arm over your head and roll onto your front for Swimming.

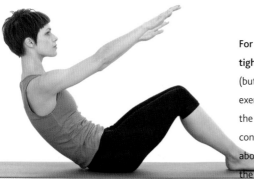

MODIFICATIONS

For a stiff lower back, back problems, tight hamstrings and weak abdominals (but also beneficial as a preparatory exercise for anybody), keep both feet on the floor and roll up and down with control, following the same instructions as above. If you need further support, hold the back of your thighs with your hands.

COMMON ERRORS

- The lifted leg lowering and sliding around
- Collapsing into the chest, with the shoulders rising to the ears
- Throwing yourself up to a sitting position from the shoulders and arms

- The abdominals bulging
- Rolling up and down with a flat back

INFORMATION

NUMBER OF REPETITIONS

3–4 on each leg.

CAUTIONS The Teaser series of exercises gets progressively harder and makes great demands on the strength of your abdominals, therefore don't proceed onto the next level before you are strong enough. For individuals with weak abdominals and lower back problems, follow the Modifications with your hands held behind your thighs, or omit the exercise. For tight hamstrings or tight lower back, it may be necessary to bend the lengthened leg; the knees should remain together.

VISUALIZATION Superglue keeps your knees together. Your chest is an air bubble, rising to the surface as you roll up.

PRECISION POINTS

- The abdominals remain hollowed throughout; they control the movement.
- The knees stay together, with the connections of the inner thigh and buttocks working to support the powerhouse.
- The shoulders press actively down the back.

Teaser I

GOALS: ✓ Strengthens the powerhouse

✓ Stabilizes the pelvis and lower trunk

✓ Trains articulation of the spine

1 **Sit on the mat, with your knees bent and legs pressed together, keeping your knees level.** Lengthen both legs so that they are extended to 45° in the Pilates stance, with your arms parallel to your legs and the back of your neck long. Balance on a slight "tuck under" of the pelvis, so that your abdominals are holding you in a C-curve.

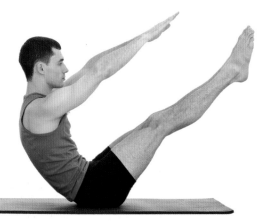

2 **Inhale and tuck your tailbone under more**, to roll back with control, with your pelvis rolling away from your legs as they remain in the same place in space. Create length as you place each vertebra on the mat.

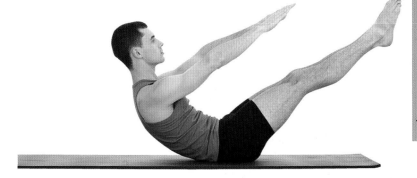

3 **Reach each of your arms overhead to the mat behind you.** Then exhale as you lift your arms forward and peel your head and spine off the mat, bone by bone, to reach your fingers toward your toes, floating up as if your upper body weighs nothing. Pause and "tease" to find your balance, with a little tuck under of your tailbone, your abdominals supporting your spine and your chest open and lifted. Inhale and roll back down, away from your legs.

TRANSITION Bend your knees and place your feet on the mat; roll down and onto your front for Swimming.

MODIFICATIONS

If Teaser I is too challenging to start with, practise Teaser I Leg (see page 192) to begin to train your strength and stamina. To progress, use the following Modification as a training tool to take you on to the full Teaser I: gently bend your knees, keeping your abdominals scooped, and roll a small way back, keeping the C-curve, then roll back up and lengthen your legs. Softly bend them again to roll back. Place your hands lightly behind the thighs if you require a little more support.

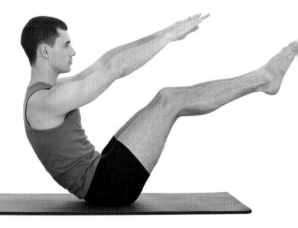

COMMON ERRORS

- The legs lowering as you roll the upper body up and down
- Losing the rib/shoulder blade connection, with the shoulders lifting to the ears and the chest sinking
- Coming back up by throwing the upper body up from the shoulders, using momentum rather than control

- Losing the scoop of the abdominals so that they protrude and the back arches

INFORMATION

NUMBER OF REPETITIONS 3.

CAUTIONS This is a very strong exercise for those with lower back issues; if not done correctly, it places stress on the spine. Use the Modifications at a level appropriate for you, or omit the exercise. For a stiff lower back, follow the Modifications for Teaser I Leg on page 194.

VISUALIZATION Your legs are so light that a helium balloon can keep them lifted. Roll your spine like a wheel.

PRECISION POINTS

- The legs are wrapped and lengthened, and don't stray from their position.
- The abdominals stay scooped and engaged.
- The spine articulates, vertebra by vertebra, on the way up and down; use control, not momentum.
- Inhale to roll back, exhale to roll up; don't breath-hold.
- The shoulders stay down the back, with the ribs in.

Swimming

✓ Lengthens the abdominals after the Teaser work

✓ Strengthens the spinal muscles in a lengthened position

✓ Teaches how to keep the abdominals working when lengthened

1 Lie on your front on the mat, with your arms and legs long, your arms as wide as your shoulders and your legs together in the centerline. Your forehead should be on the mat between your arms, with your abdominals scooped off the mat.

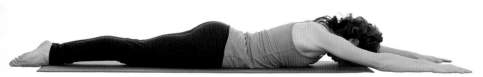

2 Inhale, lengthen as you lift your right arm and left leg, with your **head level with your right arm.** Then lengthen them even longer to lower them.

3 Exhale and lift your left arm and right leg, with your head level with **your left arm;** reach as you pause. Continue to lift and lower opposing limbs in succession.

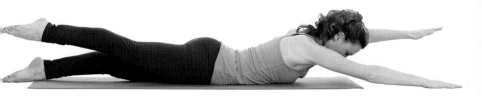

TRANSITION Push your seat back onto your heels for the Rest Position (see page 170), then stretch onto your front on the mat, ready for Leg Pull Front Support. Alternatively, place your hands on the mat under your shoulders, ready for Leg Pull Front Support.

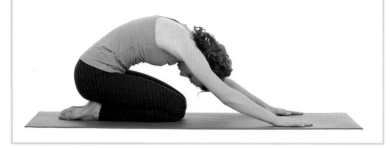

MODIFICATIONS

For tight shoulders or a tight lower back, form a diamond with your hands, place your forehead on your hands and lift alternate legs.

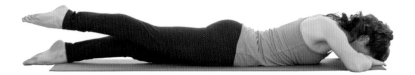

COMMON ERRORS

- The legs coming apart
- Losing the shoulder connection, with the shoulders rising to the ears and the elbows bending
- Throwing the head back and scrunching up the back of the neck
- The trunk rocking and rolling, with the pelvis lifting off the mat
- Losing the frame

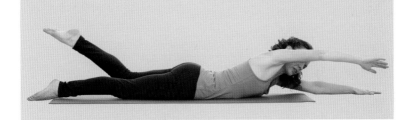

INFORMATION

NUMBER OF REPETITIONS

2–3 on each side.

CAUTIONS For shoulder injuries or tight shoulders, reduce the range of movement or follow the Modifications. For lower back pain or other back issues, proceed with caution; start with the Modifications and keep the lift of the legs low; ensure that your scoop is active throughout; omit the exercise if it is still uncomfortable on the lower back.

VISUALIZATION Lift your eyes to the horizon.

PRECISION POINTS

- The energy is on the lift!
- The pelvis stays square on the mat.
- The work is toward a lengthened, not an arched, spine.
- The shoulder blades stay engaged on the back, with long arms.

Leg Pull Front Support

GOALS: ✓ Challenges the powerhouse in a press-up position
✓ Strengthens and stabilizes the upper body

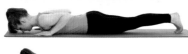

1 **Stretch out on the mat, face down.** Place your hands on the mat directly underneath your shoulders, feet flexed, with your toes under your ankles.

2 **With your legs zipped up together and your powerhouse engaged, push up to a plank position in one piece.** Breathe naturally and hold your body long and strong for a count of 10. To return to the mat: either bend your knees, lower to the floor and push your buttocks back to your heels to the Rest Position (see page 170); or lower down in one piece to the mat, in one long line.

TRANSITION Come to a kneeling position and swing your legs round to the side, so that you are sitting sideways on the mat ready for Mermaid.

MODIFICATION (A)

MODIFICATION (B)

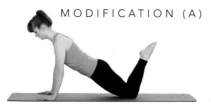

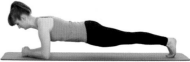

(A) Walk your hands forward on the mat from the Rest Position; lower the front of your thighs on the mat, bend your knees and bring your heels to your seat. Lengthen from your head to your knees. From the starting position, make two fists, then come onto your forearms with your elbows under your shoulders. Hook your toes under and push up into a modified plank position.
(B) To come into the full Leg Pull Front Support without pushing up from the mat, walk your hands forward on the mat from Rest Position, hook your toes under and lengthen into the Front Support position.

COMMON ERRORS

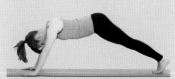

- The shoulder blades coming away from the back, so that the chest sinks and the chin pokes with an extended neck
- The hips sinking to the mat
- Losing the powerhouse, and the abdominals coming down toward the mat

INFORMATION

NUMBER OF REPETITIONS
1, with a hold for a count of 10.

CAUTIONS For weak wrists, elbows, shoulder injuries or lower back strain, exercise with care. If your powerhouse or arms are not strong enough to support you in a full plank position, then use the first Modification. If you are unable to bear weight on your wrists or hands, then either omit the exercise or use the second Modification.

VISUALIZATION Long and strong, like an arrow out of a bow.

PRECISION POINTS
- Find and maintain a strong plank shape, with the ankles, hips, knees, back and shoulders all in line.
- Don't sink between the shoulder blades: they stay strong onto the back.
- The powerhouse is visibly working—if it isn't, then gravity will take over and the stomach will sag toward the floor.

Mermaid

GOALS: ✓ Opens the ribs

✓ Stretches the sides of the spine

✓ Increases expansion in the lungs

1 **Sit sideways on your mat on your right hip, with your knees bent and your knees and ankles stacked.** Hold your ankles with your left hand; reach the other arm to the ceiling against your ear.

2 **Inhale as you lift tall out of your hips,** and reach your right hand toward the opposite wall, with your waist lengthened and your ribs opened.

3 **Exhale, lifting tall to the center,** with your arms making a T-shape.

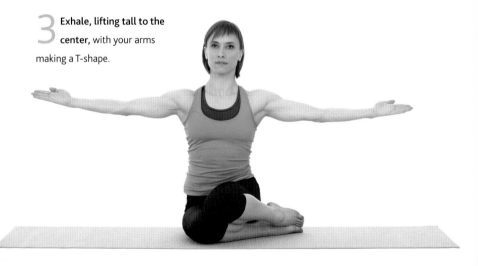

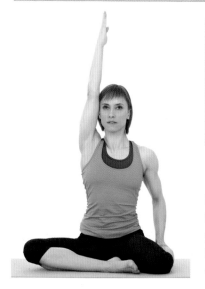

4 **Inhale and lower your right forearm to the mat, with your palm toward the ceiling.** Lengthen your left arm against your ear, and stretch toward the opposite wall; the underside of your ribs are lifted and your upper ribs opened. Exhale and, in one motion, spring back to the starting position.

TRANSITION To work the other side, come up to kneeling, reaching your arms up to the ceiling and round to the other side; sweep your feet to the opposite side and lower your hips to the mat. After completing both sides, swing your legs round to the front of the mat for Seal.

MODIFICATIONS

For tight hips, knees and general flexibility issues, separate your knees and place both legs on the mat. For knee and hip pain, use Side Stretch from the Arm-Weight Series on page 358 as a substitute.

COMMON ERRORS

- Not moving in the sideways plane of movement—that is, bending and rotating the spine.

- The arms "wafting" around; they should press strongly to the ears and are lengthened from the waist.

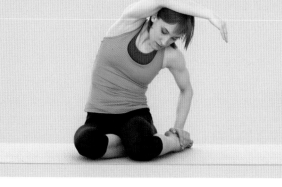

INFORMATION

NUMBER OF REPETITIONS

2–3 on each side.

CAUTIONS For tight or painful hips or knees, attempt the Modifications or omit the exercise. For shoulder problems, exercise care.

VISUALIZATION Move between two sheets of glass.

PRECISION POINTS

- The eyes are kept forward so that you remain square-on.
- The arm is pressed to the ear, not the ear to the arm, and kept there.
- The waist stays lifted throughout.
- The ribs stay flush with the body in front as they open at the sides.

Seal

GOALS:
- ✓ Used as a cool-down at the end of the mat-work
- ✓ Opens the hips in a controlled way
- ✓ Trains the powerhouse to control balance and movement

1 **Sit near the end of the mat, draw your heels in toward your seat, move your hands between your legs and place around your ankles.** Lift your feet off the floor and balance on your tailbone, scooping your powerhouse to maintain balance.

Look at your navel; your elbows should press out while your knees pull in. Your spine should be in a C-curve and your shoulders away from your ears. When you feel steady and balanced, move your legs from your hips, to clap your feet together 3 times.

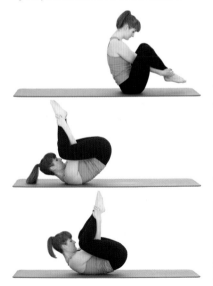

2 **Inhale and use your abdominals to support the C-curve, rolling back to the base of your shoulders.** Balance on the back of your shoulders and clap your feet together 3 times.

3 **Exhale and, using control, roll back up to your starting position.** Balance, then clap your feet together 3 times.

TRANSITION On the last repetition, release your hands, cross your ankles and reach forward to come up to a standing position. You have now completed the Intermediate Program.

MODIFICATIONS

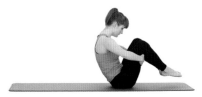

If your wrists and elbows feel vulnerable in the full position with your hands around your ankles, place your hands behind your thighs instead. If you have a tight lower back, position your hands in this alternative position.

COMMON ERRORS

- The chin tipping to the ceiling, so that the neck is strained
- Letting the knees fall out to the side
- Losing control as you roll, so that the head touches the mat as you roll back, and the feet slap the floor as you roll forward

INFORMATION

NUMBER OF REPETITIONS 6–8.

CAUTIONS If you have osteoporosis in your spine or disc problems, omit this exercise. After a hip replacement, take care with the placement of the hips, or wait until you are really strong in the hips before doing this exercise. For fragile wrists and elbows, follow the Modifications.

VISUALIZATION Clap your feet like a seal.

PRECISION POINTS

- Keep the opposition between the elbows and knees.
- Keep the chin to the chest, and the eyes to the navel.
- Use the breath to work with you in the exercise: inhale to roll back, exhale to roll up.
- At the point where you roll onto your shoulders, hold the balance as you clap your feet.

Advanced
Program

The Advanced Program greatly increases the demands for strength, stamina and coordination. The exercises grow in complexity and require that you use more challenging positions. Those exercises that you recognize from the Beginner's and Intermediate Programs become more demanding, to keep you working at your threshold.

Make sure that you are ready, add in one new move at a time, and remember: not all the moves will suit all people—there may be some moves that are not suitable for you.

The Hundred

GOALS:
- ✓ Builds on the goals of the Beginner's and Intermediate's Hundred
- ✓ Trains the strength of the powerhouse further by lowering the legs
- ✓ Uses your other connections to support the powerhouse: the wrap of the legs, ribs and shoulder blade connection
- ✓ Gets the circulation going

1 **Lie on your back, arms by your side,** and scoop your powerhouse.

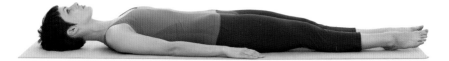

2 **Bring your knees to your chest, lift your head and lengthen your legs out at a 45° angle, with your fingers reaching long to the end of the mat.** Your scoop is pulled in, up and back, so that your spine is in contact with the mat, the tips of your shoulder blades on the mat, and you sense that your armpits are connected to your hips! Breathe in for a count of 5, then out for a count of 5, pumping your arms to the rhythm of your breath.

3 **As you warm up, lower your legs toward the mat, supported by a strong powerhouse and wrap of the legs.** The most advanced position is with your feet at eye level, but only lower your legs as far as you can while maintaining the imprint of your spine.

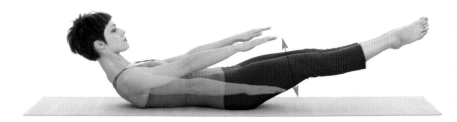

TRANSITION Bring your knees into your chest and lengthen onto the mat, ready for Roll Up.

MODIFICATIONS

The Hundred trains stamina, so you may not be ready to have your legs as low as eye level—train toward it, building up strength and stamina over time. **For a fragile neck,** place your head on a block and keep your legs toward the ceiling; omit pumping the arms if it strains your neck.

COMMON ERRORS

- Losing the connection of the upper abdominals so that the head falls back and the chin pokes to the ceiling
- Not sustaining a strong powerhouse, so that the spine is not lengthened on the mat—this can happen if you take the legs low before you are strong enough to hold them there
- The hands flapping, if the wrists aren't kept strong, with the fingers reaching away

INFORMATION

NUMBER OF REPETITIONS

100 pumps, 10 breaths.

CAUTIONS For neck and back problems, follow the beginner's exercise on page 86: use the Modifications, if necessary. If problematic shoulders are irritated by pumping the arms, keep the arms still, but lifted off the mat at hip height, reaching the fingers away.

VISUALIZATION Your body is weighted heavily into the mat.

PRECISION POINTS

- The eyes stay locked into your middle, to keep your head in the correct position.
- The ribs flatten into the waist.
- The shoulder blades "slide into your back pockets."
- Imprint the spine from the tip of the tailbone to the base of the shoulder blades.
- Wrap the legs in the Pilates stance and lengthen out of the hips.
- The trunk stays still and stable as you pump the arms.

Roll Up

GOALS:
- ✓ Creates a dynamic stretch to the hamstrings and the muscles along the back of the body
- ✓ Trains the powerhouse to be strong and active throughout the whole range of spinal motion
- ✓ Teaches articulation of the vertebrae, and control of movement of individual vertebra using the abdominal muscles

1 Lie on the mat, zipped up strongly into your centerline, with your legs pressed together and feet flexed. Reach your arms overhead, with your elbows by your ears.

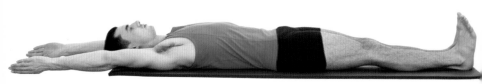

2 Inhale and lift your chin to your chest to initiate rolling up; as you do so, bring your arms up, so that your head stays between your arms. As you start to roll up, funnel your ribs further and pull your abdominals in deeper to your spine. Roll up off the mat, one bone at a time.

3 Exhale, reaching your hands beyond your toes. Your powerhouse is strongly pulled in, up and back, to keep your abdominals lifted away from your thighs, creating a C-curve from the crown of your head to your tailbone. Create a sense of opposition as your fingers reach forward and your powerhouse lifts up and back into the spine.

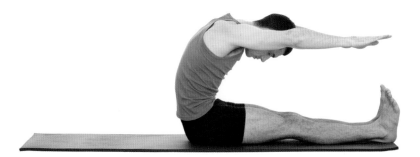

4 **Inhale, using your abdominals; tuck your tailbone under to articulate your spine—sacrum first, then lower back, then waist.** Exhale as your powerhouse controls your descent onto the mat, bone by bone, until you are lying on it. Take your arms overhead, but don't lose your scoop or your rib connection in the lengthened position. With the next inhalation, begin again, keeping the move fluid—this will help train your stamina!

> **TRANSITION**
> Lie in the center of the mat, ready for Roll Over.

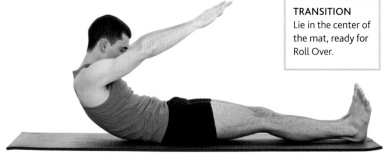

MODIFICATIONS

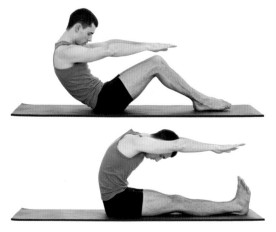

For a tight, stiff lower back, keep your knees bent as you roll back up. As you reach your arms, lengthen your legs, then bend them again to roll back.

COMMON ERRORS

- The spine arching, with the ribs flailing and the abdominals bulging
- Chin poking forward

- Losing the centerline connection of the legs
- Not articulating the spine, and lowering down with a flat back
- Using the shoulders to throw yourself up off the mat

INFORMATION

NUMBER OF REPETITIONS 5.

CAUTIONS For a stiff lower back, use the modified intermediate version on page 134. For lower back pain, use the beginner's version Roll Down on page 90, or omit altogether. For disc problems, do Roll Down on page 90 with caution, or omit.

VISUALIZATION Your spine is a wheel that rolls up and down in one continuous motion.

PRECISION POINTS

- The legs are kept pulled together strongly from the heels to the seat.
- Keep the legs firmly on the mat by reaching them away from you, as you roll up and down.
- As you bend forward to reach your toes, don't let your chest collapse onto your thighs—keep the spine lifted.
- The ribs and abdominals are kept engaged throughout the move; as you take your arms over your head, maintain the rib/shoulder blade connection, and keep the back of the ribs imprinted on the mat.

Roll Over

GOALS: ✓ Lengthens out the spinal muscles

✓ Articulates the spine

✓ Increases flexibility of the spine, hamstrings, calf muscles and shoulders

✓ Works the lower abdominals

1 **Lie on the mat, with your legs pressed together toward the ceiling and perpendicular to the floor,** arms by your side and neck lengthened.

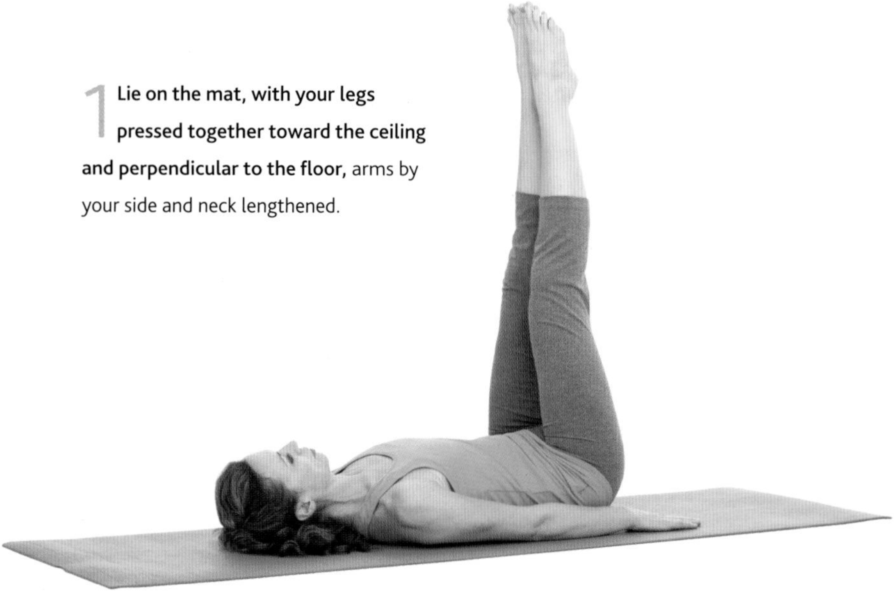

2 Inhale and, lifting from your lower abdominals and backside, take your legs overhead until they are parallel to the floor. Press your palms into the mat to keep your arms long, with your throat soft and shoulders open.

3 Flex your feet to reach through your heels, and open your legs to hip-width apart. The back of your neck stays long, as the weight is on the back of your shoulders.

4 **Exhale and initiate rolling down, by slowly reversing the articulation of each bone of your spine onto the mat.** Your powerhouse and backside should control the descent slowly, keeping your legs close to your body so that they follow the spine down, until the tailbone arrives on the mat and the legs are at a 90° angle

again. Then close the legs and inhale to lift again. After the third repetition, keep your legs hip-width apart to lift up and over, then close them when they are overhead and repeat 3 times. To progress, take your feet to the floor when the legs are overhead and flex the feet further. As you lower your legs to the starting position, take them a little beyond the 90° angle, maintaining the imprint of your spine using your powerhouse.

TRANSITION From the starting position, lengthen your left leg to the mat and keep your right leg reaching through the heel to the ceiling, in a slight Pilates stance, ready for One-Leg Circles.

MODIFICATIONS

For back problems, omit this exercise.
If you have tight hamstrings and a stiff lower back, you may need to omit this exercise until your flexibility has improved.

COMMON ERRORS

- Letting the weight fall onto the neck
- Letting gravity take the legs so that they fall over your head
- The abdominals bulging as you lower the legs
- Using momentum to hoist the legs overhead
- Lowering the spine down in one block
- The shoulders rising so that the elbows and wrists bend

INFORMATION

NUMBER OF REPETITIONS

3 in each direction.

CAUTIONS Omit this exercise for back and neck problems. Proceed with caution with some shoulder issues. Be aware of your own flexibility, as it may limit your ability to do this exercise without straining your back, neck or shoulders.

VISUALIZATION Pop a grape with each vertebra as you place each bone back on the mat. Your arms are strapped to the mat along their whole length.

PRECISION POINTS

- The weight is on the shoulders, not the neck.
- Work to a strong centerline and peel off and replace the spine along an imaginary line on the mat.
- The palms stay pressed into the mat.
- As you roll down, reach through the heels to feel opposition between the legs and the spine, with the legs close to the body.
- Move smoothly and with control.

One-Leg Circles

GOALS: ✓ Improves flexibility of the hamstrings and iliotibial band

✓ Helps maintain alignment at the hip, knee, pelvis and spine while moving the leg

✓ The bigger movement of the leg provides an even greater challenge to stability than the beginner's and intermediate versions, increasing the difficulty and intensity of the exercise

✓ Frees up the hip

1 **Lie on the mat and reach your right leg toward the ceiling with a slight turn-out into the Pilates stance.** Your toes should be in line with your nose; your left leg reaches long onto the mat, strong into your centerline. Your spine should be lengthened on the mat.

2 **Inhale and move your right leg long across your body to the opposite shoulder,** stabilizing with a strong powerhouse.

3 **Circle your leg down,** continuing to reach it long.

4 **Exhale and bring your leg out, then whip it back up to the starting position.** The emphasis is on the up! Repeat 5 times, then reverse the circles.

5 **Scissors your legs in mid-air to change legs;** repeat with the left leg.

TRANSITION Lengthen both legs on the mat, then lift your arms to the ceiling, chin to your chest. Roll up to a sitting position, articulating your spine as you come up. Bring yourself forward on the mat for Rolling Like a Ball.

MODIFICATIONS

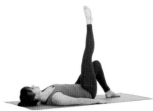

If you have a tight neck, shoulders or hamstrings, or difficulties with your back or neck, then keep the other leg bent with the foot flat on the mat. Refer to the beginner's or intermediate versions on pages 94 and 136, using the Modifications if necessary.

COMMON ERRORS

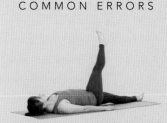

- Losing the length in the back of the neck and letting the chin lift to the ceiling
- Not using the powerhouse to stabilize the spine and pelvis on the mat
- Losing the length in the lifted leg, so that the knee is soggy

INFORMATION

NUMBER OF REPETITIONS
5 times each way on each leg.

CAUTIONS For back problems, refer to the beginner's exercise on page 94. For clicking hips, reduce the range of motion at the hip and wrap the seat and inner thigh.

VISUALIZATION Draw a large perfect circle in the air with your toe.

PRECISION POINTS
- Soften and broaden the collarbone to keep the chest open.
- Reach one leg long to the ceiling and the other away on the mat, with a strong anchor in the middle.
- The spine stays imprinted; the movement of the leg should not cause the spine and pelvis to shift.
- The progression is in creating larger circles, but maintaining stability.
- The move is dynamic—get it moving!

Rolling Like a Ball

GOALS: ✓ Trains the abdominal muscles in strength and control

✓ Massages the spine and opens up the back muscles

✓ Teaches alignment and moving with symmetry

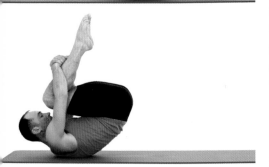

1 **Balance on your sit-bones at the front of the mat, knees slightly apart, feet in a Pilates point.** Wrap your hands in front of your ankles, with one hand holding the opposite wrist. Keep your heels in toward your backside. Lift from your powerhouse as you bring your chin to your chest and your forehead between your knees. You are now the shape of a ball!

2 **Inhale and, initiating from the abdominals, roll back, keeping yourself pulled in tight to your ball shape and your centerline.** Roll to the tip of your shoulder blades. Exhale, pull your abdominals in deeper and roll up to the point of balance. Pause and find the balance on your tailbone, then inhale and roll back again.

TRANSITION From the balance, pull your right knee in, place your right hand to your right shin and your left hand to your right knee, then reach your left leg away from you with a straight knee. Roll down to the mat in this shape for Single Leg Stretch.

MODIFICATIONS

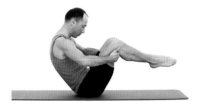

If you have knee problems, take your hands behind your thighs—see the beginner's version on page 98.

COMMON ERRORS

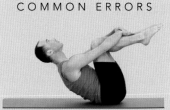

- Throwing the head back to initiate the rolling
- Losing the C-curve, and rolling with a flat back
- Losing the connection between the heels and the seat
- Using the biceps to pull yourself back up

INFORMATION

NUMBER OF REPETITIONS 6–8.

CAUTIONS For osteoporosis, omit any rolling exercises if you have bone-density problems more severe than osteopenia. If you have a significant scoliosis, omit this exercise. For back problems, exercise caution; if you have disc problems, omit this exercise. If you have knee problems, hold behind the thigh.

VISUALIZATION Roll like a coin rolling on its edge.

PRECISION POINTS

- Stay in the shape of a ball.
- Do not pull up using your arms—use your abdominals.
- Roll only to the base of the shoulders, not the head and neck.
- Keep the lower back lifted into the C-curve throughout.
- Keep the heels to the seat, forehead between the knees, and shoulders down the back.

Abdominal Five Series: Single Leg Stretch

GOALS:
- ✓ Trains stamina in the abdominals
- ✓ Trains many connections simultaneously: the powerhouse, centerline, ribs/shoulder blades
- ✓ Challenges greater stabilization of the trunk, with movement of all the limbs

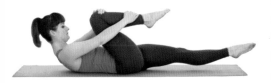

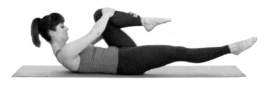

TRANSITION Draw both knees into your chest and, holding your ankles, keep your head up, ready for Double Leg Stretch.

1 Lie in the center of the mat, head up, right knee drawn in and in line with the right shoulder; your right hand is on your ankle, left hand on your right knee. The left leg should lengthen as low as possible, maintaining the imprint of your spine on the mat, with your lower abdominals deeply scooped.

2 Inhale and change legs. Pull your left leg in strongly, and lengthen your right leg out parallel with the mat, or as low as you can take it. Exhale and change legs. Reach out long, to pull in strong! Move with a strong, dynamic rhythm, centering your body along your midline.

MODIFICATIONS

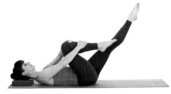

If you have difficulties with your neck, or if it fatigues, place your head on a block, refer to the Modification in the intermediate version on page 143 and keep the extended leg at a 45° angle. **If you have knee problems,** place your hands behind your thighs and avoid pressing on the knee joint. **If you have a weak or vulnerable back,** refer to the Modification in the beginner's version on page 103.

COMMON ERRORS

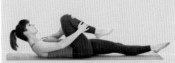

- Extended the lowered leg below the level of the hip, with the lower abdominals losing the scoop so that the abdominals bulge
- The legs losing their centerline connection
- Losing the rib/shoulder blade connection so that the shoulders lift
- The tailbone curling off the mat

INFORMATION

NUMBER OF REPETITIONS 6–10.

CAUTIONS For knee, neck and back issues, refer to the Modifications.

VISUALIZATION The area from your tailbone to the base of your shoulder blades has grown roots into the mat. Imagine your heels sliding on an imaginary sheet of glass to keep the centerline.

PRECISION POINTS
- The extended leg is lengthened, level with the hip.
- The abdominals are lifted to create a strong center.
- Keep the ribs in, the shoulder blades down your back and the elbows lifted, to create a strong diamond with the arms.

Abdominal Five Series: Double Leg Stretch

GOALS:
- ✓ Builds from the intermediate level on the challenge of training strength and stamina in the abdominals
- ✓ Challenges further the sense of opposition in two directions from a strong center
- ✓ Coordinates the breath between the powerhouse and the movement

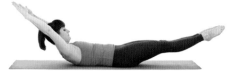

1 **Lie on your mat, use your powerhouse to draw your knees into your chest.** Hold your ankles, with your knees slightly parted. Ensure that your tailbone is on the mat with your spine imprinted, and your head is up, with your eyes on your navel.

2 **Inhale and reach your limbs out long in opposite directions.** With your arms by your ears; your legs should lengthen in the Pilates stance. Keep your eyes on your navel, with your powerhouse pulled in deeply, and your spine and ribs firmly imprinted on the mat.

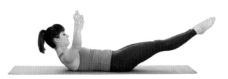

3 **Exhale and take the arms out and round,** as you pull your knees into your chest from a strong center, hugging them as you squeeze the last drop of air out of your lungs.

TRANSITION Take both legs to the ceiling; hold the right ankle ready for Single Straight-Leg Stretch 'Scissors'.

MODIFICATIONS

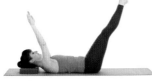

If you struggle to keep your head up, use a block under it and bring your legs toward the ceiling more.

COMMON ERRORS

- Losing the rib/shoulder blade connection so that the ribs flare, the shoulders lift to the ears and the chin pokes out
- The abdominals bulging as the limbs lengthen
- Tucking the tailbone under

INFORMATION

NUMBER OF REPETITIONS 6–10.

CAUTIONS For knee pain, bring the hands behind the thighs, not to the ankles or shins. For shoulder problems, limit the range of motion by lifting the arms toward the ceiling and bringing the hands just to the ankles. For back and neck problems, proceed with caution and refer to the modified beginner's version on page 106.

VISUALIZATION Imagine yourself lengthening like elastic as you stretch.

PRECISION POINTS

- Keep the ribs flush to the front and the shoulder blades sliding down the back.
- The powerhouse is pulled in and up, to maintain the imprint of the spine.
- The tailbone stays glued to the mat on drawing the limbs in.
- The legs are wrapped as they lengthen.

Abdominal Five Series: Single Straight-Leg Stretch 'Scissors'

GOALS: ✓ Trains strength and stamina in the abdominals
✓ Challenges the flexibility of the hamstrings

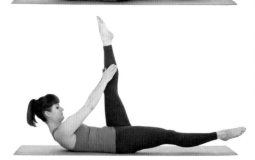

1 **Lie on the mat with both legs flat on the floor, then take the right leg up and stretch the other leg away.** Hold your right ankle with both hands and pull it toward you for a double pulse. Your spine should stay lengthened on the mat from the tailbone to the base of your shoulder blades. Your elbows should be wide and lifted, with the ribs and shoulder blades engaged.

2 **Switch legs in a scissor-like motion and pulse-pulse.** To progress, bring the leg in for a single pulse. The rhythm should be strong and dynamic—keep it moving! Inhale for one repetition (both legs scissored); exhale for the next.

TRANSITION Take both legs toward the ceiling and both hands behind the head, ready for Double Straight-Leg Stretch. If you need to rest your neck, lower your head briefly.

MODIFICATIONS

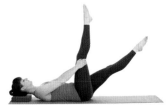

For tight hamstrings and lack of flexibility, place your hands on your leg so that you can maintain the imprint of your spine as you bring the leg in. Keep the range of movement of your legs smaller. For a weak neck, use a block under your head.

COMMON ERRORS

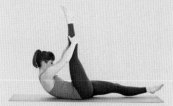

- The whole shoulders lifting off the mat, so that the body is in a curled-up position
- Losing the energy and work in the legs, so that the knees bend
- The powerhouse not stabilizing the trunk, so that it rolls as the legs move

INFORMATION

NUMBER OF REPETITIONS
6–10 on each leg.

CAUTIONS If the neck fatigues, rest it intermittently.

VISUALIZATION Cut the air with the blades of the scissors, as your legs move through space.

PRECISION POINTS
- The lower leg reaches away long and strong on the centerline; the legs are in a Pilates stance.
- The tips of the shoulder blades are kept on the mat; don't let the shoulders roll off the mat.
- The box shape is maintained.
- The legs move from the powerhouse.

Abdominal Five Series: Double Straight-Leg Stretch 'Lower Lifts'

GOALS: ✓ Trains control and strength in the powerhouse

✓ Challenges stamina in the powerhouse

1 **Lie on the mat with both legs flat on the floor.** Raise your head and take both legs to the ceiling in the Pilates stance. Place your hands behind your head, with one hand laid over the other. Keep your elbows within your line of vision and your eyes locked on your middle. Your powerhouse should be very active, with your spine firmly on the mat from your tailbone to the base of your shoulder blades.

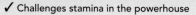

2 **Inhale and lower your legs away from you,** for a count of 1.

3 **Keep scooped and lower the legs further,** for a count of 2.

4 **For a count of 3** maintain the imprint of the spine and lower your legs as far as you can. Exhale and let your legs spring back to the starting position.

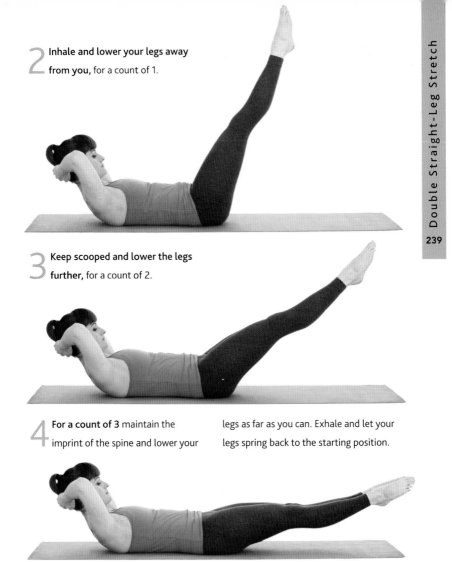

TRANSITION Bring your right knee in to your chest and lengthen your left leg long, in line with your nose. Your hands should stay behind your head, ready for Criss-Cross.

MODIFICATIONS

If your powerhouse isn't strong enough to maintain your spine on the mat while your legs lower, or your hamstrings are tight, adopt one of the following modifications:

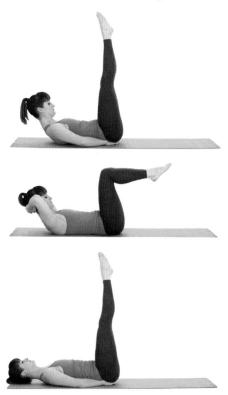

(A) Keep your head up, make a diamond shape with your hands and place them under your tailbone. Keep the movement of your legs smaller.

(B) Keep your head up, with your hands behind your head and your knees bent at a 90° angle in a tabletop position. Only lower your legs a small distance from the body.

(C) For neck problems, keep your head on the mat, make a diamond shape with your hands and place them under your tailbone.

COMMON ERRORS

- The ribs and belly losing the scoop and bulging
- Lowering the legs too far, so that the abdominals cannot take the weight

- of the legs, causing the back to lift off the mat
- The tailbone rolling up off the mat when lifting the legs

INFORMATION

NUMBER OF REPETITIONS 6–10.

CAUTIONS If you have back problems, omit this exercise. For weak abdominals, proceed with caution: either use the Modifications or omit this exercise until you are strong enough. If you have neck problems, use Modification C.

VISUALIZATION Paint an arc on the wall in front with your toes.

PRECISION POINTS

- The spine must *not* lose contact with the mat at any stage of the exercise.
- The tailbone stays plugged into the mat as the legs come up to the perpendicular.
- The abdominals, not the hands, keep the head up, so the elbows should stay wide.
- The legs are long and strong, with a wrap around the buttocks to help support the powerhouse.

Abdominal Five Series: Criss-Cross

GOALS: ✔ Strengthens and increases stamina in the abdominals

✔ Specifically works the oblique abdominal muscles

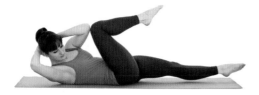

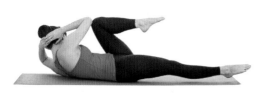

TRANSITION Lengthen your legs on the mat, with your hands toward the ceiling, and roll up ready for Spine Stretch Forward.

1 **Lie on the mat with both legs flat on the floor, hands behind the head.** Inhale and bring the right knee in, so that it is in line with the right shoulder. Lift the upper body and twist, so that your left elbow and right knee touch. Your abdominals should lift your upper body, so that your shoulders are clear of the mat. Your right elbow reaches back and your eyes should follow it; the elbow stays lifted off the mat.

2 **Exhale, keep your upper body lifted high and change sides, with your left leg in and left knee touching your right elbow.** Your eyes should be on the left elbow as it reaches back.

MODIFICATIONS

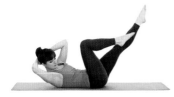

For a weaker back or abdominals, take the lengthened leg toward the ceiling.

COMMON ERRORS

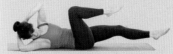

- The hands pulling on the neck, with the elbows dropping in and the shoulders lifting to the ears
- Losing the work from the upper abdominals, so that the shoulders lower to the mat as you switch sides
- Losing the 'box' on the mat, so that the trunk is rocking around

INFORMATION

NUMBER OF REPETITIONS 6–10.

CAUTIONS For weak necks or neck problems, omit this exercise. Due to the rotation in this exercise, proceed with caution for back injuries; it may be necessary to omit this exercise.

VISUALIZATION The hips and spine, from the tailbone to the upper middle back, sink into wet sand.

PRECISION POINTS
There is huge potential to steam through this exercise, but without focusing on the Precision points you won't feel the benefits; do it properly and you will reap the rewards:

- Maintain a steady rhythm—resist the temptation to race through, and hold onto the lift to each side.
- The upper abdominals work hard to maintain the lift of the shoulders throughout.
- Keep the pelvis and lower back imprinted on the mat.
- Keep the box square, and work to a strong centerline, so that the legs stay within the frame.
- The heels reach to the same point.

Spine Stretch Forward

GOALS:
✓ Develops flexibility in the hamstrings
✓ Teaches you how to sit tall and lift out of the hips
✓ Articulates the spine

1 **Sit on the mat with your legs straight and just wider than mat-width apart.** Use your powerhouse and your seat muscles to sit tall and lift out of your hips. Lift your arms to shoulder height, parallel to the floor and shoulder-width apart, with the palms facing down. As you work your backside muscles, you will gain height and a sense of being lifted and lengthened through the crown of your head. You will feel as if you are very active in your pelvic floor, backside and abdominal muscles.

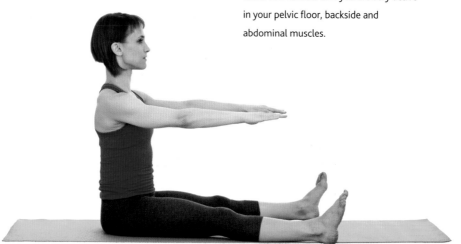

2 **Exhale,** put your chin to your chest and lift your abdominals as you roll the spine down.

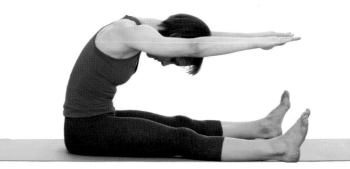

3 **Work the crown of your head toward the mat, to create a capital C-shape; your bottom ribs should lift in and up to deepen the curve.** Feel a deep stretch as your fingers reach forward and your powerhouse lifts your spine, your toes face the ceiling and you reach through your heels. Exhale completely. Inhale and reverse the articulation, using your abdominals to roll up, one vertebra at a time, so that you are sitting tall with your shoulders over your hips.

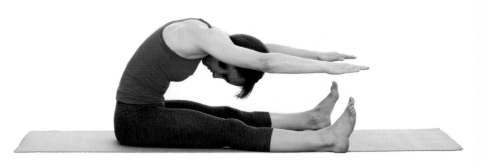

TRANSITION Lift again to reach for your ankles and draw your heels in toward you, ready for Open-Leg Rocker.

MODIFICATIONS

For flexibility issues with your hamstrings or lower back, use a block so that you can sit tall with your shoulders over your hips; or softly bend your knees (see the beginner's version and the Modifications on pages 108–9).

For painful shoulders, slide your hands on the mat between your legs.

COMMON ERRORS

- The toes and knees rolling in
- Bending from the hips with a flat back, and not creating a C-curve in the spine
- Palms turning toward the floor, with the shoulders sliding up to the ears

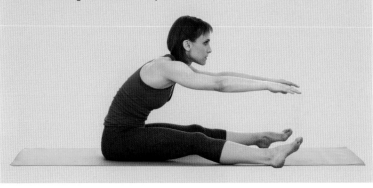

INFORMATION

NUMBER OF REPETITIONS 5.

CAUTIONS For low back and shoulder problems, follow the Modifications, or the modified beginner's version on page 109.

VISUALIZATION Create a large capital C, with the head working the top of the C to the mat.

PRECISION POINTS

- The toes and knees face the ceiling.
- Create a lifted "round" in the spine, not a flat back.
- Stack the spine to roll back up; don't come up in one movement, with a flat back.
- Keep your backside muscles active throughout, to keep the sensation of being lifted.

Open-Leg Rocker

GOALS: ✓ Trains the powerhouse and the body in control, balance and coordination

✓ Develops flexibility of the spine and hamstrings

✓ Massages the spine

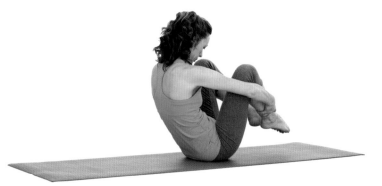

1 **Sit on the mat and take hold of the outside of your ankles and bring your heels in.** Tip back and balance on your tailbone, with your knees shoulder-width apart and your toes soft.

2 **Lengthen out both legs, keeping the back of your neck lengthened and your chest lifted.** This a challenging balance: when you are there, you will feel that there is a little point on which you are able to maintain the balance, with your scoop working hard, lifting and supporting your spine, with opposing energy through the top of your head and your legs.

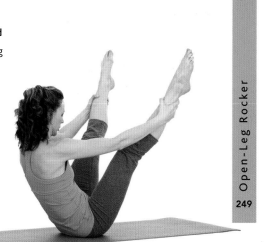

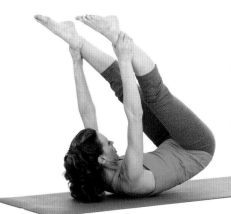

3 **Inhale and, with your eyes on your navel, roll back, initiating the roll from your abdominals.** Then exhale and roll back up, pulling your abdominals in. Pause and find the balance at the top, with your chest lifted; your eyes should find the horizon.

MODIFICATIONS

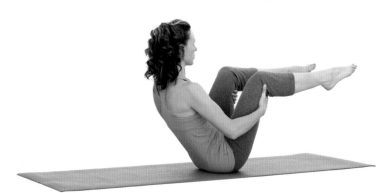

For tight hamstrings and general flexibility issues, adjust your hand position; aim to have it as few places as possible away from your ankles, so that you are working toward the ideal of the exercise. If you have very tight hamstrings, hold behind the thighs and bend your knees, so that your lower legs are parallel to the floor, and simply balance there.

TRANSITION Close your legs, release your hands from your ankles and, with control, roll your body down away from your legs, until your back is on the mat and your legs are perpendicular, ready for Corkscrew II.

COMMON ERRORS

- The chest collapses, allowing the chin to poke forward
- Losing the connection of the shoulder blades, so that they elevate toward the ears and protract forward
- The legs fall outside the frame
- Rolling onto the head and neck

- Bending the knees to help with the roll-up
- Using the arms and pulling on the legs to come up

INFORMATION

NUMBER OF REPETITIONS 6–8.

CAUTIONS For tender tailbones, it may be too uncomfortable to proceed. For disc and other recent back injuries, omit this exercise. For problems with flexibility, or if you are not yet strong enough for the exercise, follow the Modifications.

VISUALIZATION Roll like a skateboarder on a semicircular ramp; pause at the top, then roll again.

PRECISION POINTS
- In the balance, keep the eyes on the horizon with the chest lifted.
- Keep the eyes on the navel.
- The spine stays lifted throughout, from an active powerhouse.
- Rolling is only onto the shoulders.

Corkscrew II

GOALS: ✓ Cultivates stability in the trunk

✓ Trains strength in the lower abdominals

✓ Teaches how to move the legs separately from the pelvis

1 Lie on your back on the mat, with your legs pointing directly to the ceiling, wrapped in the centerline. Your arms should rest with your palms on the mat and the back of your shoulders in contact with the mat, so that your chest is softly open. Inhale and take the legs, as one, across to your left hip, then circle the legs down and to the center, maintaining the imprint of your spine on the mat. Exhale and complete the circle, with your powerhouse scooped strongly into your spine.

2 As you return your legs to the center, peel your pelvis and your lowest four or five vertebrae off the mat and lift your legs toward the ceiling. Then lower your spine down with control, one vertebra at a time. Reverse the circle, and repeat the lift.

TRANSITION
Bring your legs together in the center, raise your hands to the ceiling and come up in one movement for Saw.

MODIFICATIONS

If you are not strong enough for this exercise at present, work on Corkscrew I on page 162. **For tight hamstrings and a weak back,** follow the Modification for Corkscrew I on page 164.

COMMON ERRORS

- Losing the length of the spine on the mat, with the lower back lifting and the chin poking toward the ceiling
- The shoulders popping forward
- Losing the centerline connection of the legs so that one heel moves forward of the other
- The weight bearing through the neck, rather than through the shoulders and body

INFORMATION

NUMBER OF REPETITIONS
2–4 in each direction.

CAUTIONS For a weak neck, proceed with caution; do not allow weight to bear on the neck during the move. For a recent back injury, omit this exercise. If you are not strong enough for the lift, continue to work at Corkscrew I on page 162 until you are strong enough.

VISUALIZATION Use the feet to draw an imaginary circle, then lift the feet up through the center of that circle.

PRECISION POINTS
- The collarbone remain softened and open.
- The connection of the ribs and shoulders are used to keep firm contact with the mat.
- The legs move as one.
- The roll-down is controlled, with the neck remaining long and the shoulders on the mat.

Saw

✓ Trains the powerhouse to lift the spine and rotate
✓ Works the oblique abdominals in a sitting position

1 **Sit tall on the mat with an active powerhouse and backside to lift you out of your hips with an elongated spine.** Your legs should be long and just wider than the mat, with your feet flexed and your heels reaching away in front. Lift your arms to shoulder height out to the sides, but keep them in the periphery of your vision. When you are correctly set up, you should feel tall and lifted through your center, with your energy reaching three ways: through the top of your head, through your heels and through your fingertips.

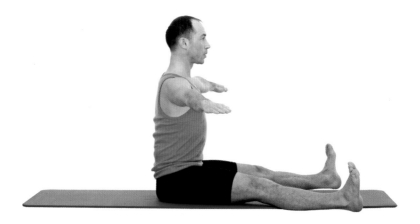

2 **Inhale to lift your spine more,** and twist from your waist to the right.

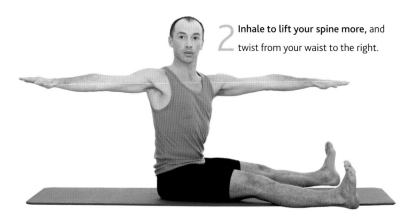

3 **Exhale and reach your left little finger past your right little toe; your right hand reaches up and back, with the palm facing the ceiling.** "Saw" the little finger past the toe for a count of 1, 2, then reach even further for 3, wringing the air out of your lungs. The twist and the reach come from your powerhouse, with your front and back hands reaching away in opposition. Repeat on the other side.

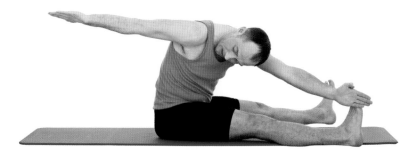

TRANSITION Your arms and legs come together to the
center . Then roll down and onto your front for Swan Dive.

MODIFICATIONS

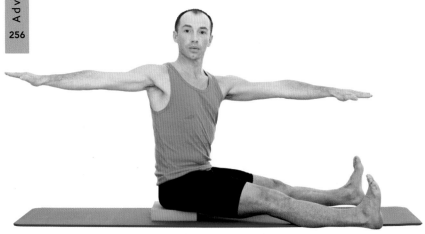

For tight hamstrings and lower back, sit
on a block. **For shoulder and back issues,**
refer to the Modification in the beginner's
version on page 112.

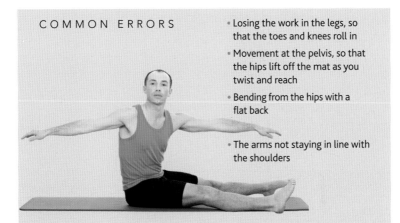

COMMON ERRORS

- Losing the work in the legs, so that the toes and knees roll in
- Movement at the pelvis, so that the hips lift off the mat as you twist and reach
- Bending from the hips with a flat back
- The arms not staying in line with the shoulders

Saw

257

INFORMATION

NUMBER OF REPETITIONS 3–5.

CAUTIONS For shoulder problems that are irritated by the combination of elevation and reach, follow the modified beginner's version on page 112, or omit the exercise. For back issues, particularly disc problems, use the modified beginner's version, or omit altogether, due to the combination of bend and twist.

VISUALIZATION "Saw" off your little toe as you reach.

PRECISION POINTS

- The heels stay level as you reach past the little toe; if one moves forward of the other, then your pelvis has shifted.
- The toes and knees remain facing the ceiling.
- The spine is in a C-curve as you reach.
- Each time you twist, lift more out of the hips.
- The hand that reaches back has the palm facing the ceiling, and your eyes follow the back arm.
- The shoulders stay down the back.

Swan Dive Preparation and Swan Dive

GOALS: ✓ Lengthens and strengthens the spine

✓ Works the abdominals in a lengthened position

SWAN DIVE PREPARATION

1 **Lie face down on the mat, with your forehead in contact with the mat,** hands under your shoulders, elbows pulled tightly into your ribs, and your shoulder blades actively working down your back. Your legs should be zipped up together in the centerline, from the heels to the seat.

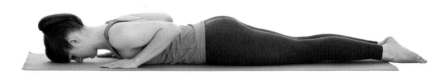

2 **Inhale, lift your abdominals in and lengthen your upper body off the mat.** Your eyes should be directed to the horizon, and your chest lifted and open. There should be equal pressure on both hands, with your elbows pressed into your side.

3 **Exhale and, working your elbows into your sides, lift your hands 1 inch (2.5 cm) off the mat, and dive forward.** Stay pressed into your centerline, with your legs and back working strongly; your legs should lift to the ceiling, as you form the shape of a banana in the dive. Inhale, pressing your hands into the mat, lifting your eyes to the horizon and maintaining the same shape in space. Dive 3–5 times, without pausing at either end of the dive.

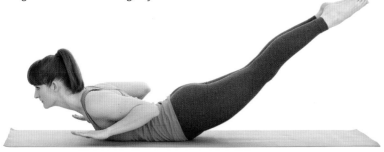

If you are able to carry out Swan Dive Preparation with no adverse reactions, then you are ready for the full Swan Dive. Warm up either by doing the Swan Neck Roll on page 168 or by lifting and lowering your upper body 2–3 times.

4 **Set up in the same way as for steps 1 and 2.** Inhale and take your hands from the mat, then lift your arms in one motion up in front of you, in line with your ears, with your palms facing one another; dive forward, with your legs lifting toward the ceiling.

5 **Exhale and dive;** to lift the chest and arms toward the ceiling, keep the shape in your body so as your upper body lifts, your legs lower toward the mat. Dive back and forth 3–5 times: inhale to dive forward, exhale to lift the chest. Keep it moving.

TRANSITION Lying face down on the mat, make two fists and draw your elbows in strongly, so that you are supported, but lifted on both forearms, ready for Single Leg Kicks.

MODIFICATIONS

This is a very strong exercise; if you are not ready for it, follow the Swan Neck Roll on page 168.

COMMON ERRORS

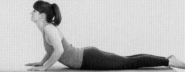

- Losing the centerline connection
- Not moving from the powerhouse so the tummy bulges and the chin protrudes
- Using the arms too much, with the shoulders rising toward the ears
- Throwing the head back, and straining the neck
- Losing the shape you have created, with the head moving separately from the rest of the spine, like a bobbing duck rather than an elegant swan

INFORMATION

NUMBER OF REPETITIONS 3–5.

CAUTIONS For back injuries and related issues, omit this exercise. For wrist, elbow, shoulder and neck issues, proceed with caution. Start with the Swan Neck Roll on page 168, and use it to prepare for the stronger move of Swan Dive Preparation.

VISUALIZATION You are the rockers on a rocking chair: rock back and forth, in a smooth arc.

PRECISION POINTS

- The legs and backside are kept active.
- It is paramount to keep the abdominals active throughout, to avoid the spine feeling pinched.
- The elbows reach to the heels, with the shoulders engaged.
- This is a dynamic exercise—there is no reduced pace; dive forward to dive up!

Single Leg Kicks

GOALS:
- ✓ Stretches the front of the thighs and hips
- ✓ Trains stability of the shoulders, and tones the upper arms
- ✓ Strengthens the muscles along the back of the body
- ✓ Challenges the powerhouse, in a lengthened position

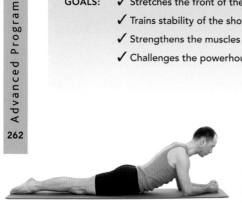

1 **Lie on your front on the mat, make two fists and pull them strongly toward you, so that you are propped on your forearms, which are pressed into the mat.** Your eyes should be on the horizon, your neck long and your pelvis on the mat. Your legs are zipped up, with your shoulders sliding down your back; your chest is lifted, and your abdominals are working.

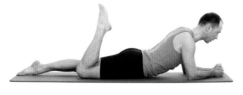

2 **Inhale and kick your right heel to your right buttock,** with a double pulse: kick-kick.

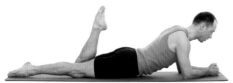

3 **Switch your legs in space.** Your right leg lengthens to the mat as the left pulses: kick-kick. Exhale and repeat.

TRANSITION Lengthen down on your front, turn your head to the right and bring your hands together behind your back, ready for Double Leg Kicks.

MODIFICATIONS

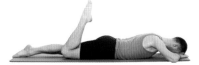

Make a diamond shape with both hands, place your forehead on the diamond and follow the instructions opposite, with your head down.

C O M M O N   E R R O R S

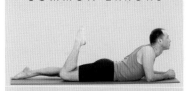

- The chest sinking, the chin poking out and the shoulder blades popping
- The lower back collapsing, with the stomach sagging to the mat
- The pelvis lifting off the mat or rocking around

263

INFORMATION

NUMBER OF REPETITIONS
3–5 on each leg.

CAUTIONS For lower back issues, weak abdominals or tight hips/quadriceps, follow the Modifications. For knee issues, either omit the exercise or limit the range of motion and decrease the pace, so that the move is pain-free.

VISUALIZATION Your head is as light as a helium balloon, keeping the rest of your spine lifted.

PRECISION POINTS
- The forearms are pressed into the mat with a strong powerhouse, to keep the spine lifted and long.
- The elbows are under the shoulders.
- The heels kick to the center of the buttocks.
- The legs have a centerline connection, and the pelvis presses into the mat.
- There is a dynamic pattern of kick-kick-switch.

Double Leg Kicks

GOALS:
- ✓ Opens the front of the chest
- ✓ Brings flexibility to the spine and shoulders
- ✓ Strengthens the muscles along the back of the body
- ✓ Challenges the powerhouse, in a lengthened position

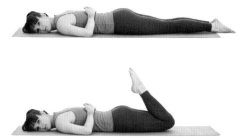

1 **Lie on your front, with your head turned to the left.** Place one hand over the other high up your back, with your palms facing the ceiling and your elbows to the mat. Your legs should be pressed strongly into the centerline, with your powerhouse pulled in and your pelvis pressed into the mat.

2 **Inhale and kick both legs to your buttocks promptly,** 3 times.

3 **Lengthen your legs to the mat.** Exhale as your hands lift and reach long toward your heels to pull your upper body up, with your eyes to the horizon and your chest open. Lengthen for a count of 3. Then turn your head to the right and lower your upper body to the mat. Repeat; inhale with the kick, exhale with the lift.

TRANSITION Push your backside onto your heels in the Rest Position (see page 170). Place your palms down to one side, lift your hips to one side and roll onto your back, ready for Neck Pull.

MODIFICATIONS

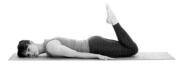

For tight shoulders, work with your arms by your sides, palms down.

COMMON ERRORS

- During the leg kicks the pelvis pops off the mat and the elbows lift
- Legs losing the centerline connection
- Legs lifting as the upper body lifts, creating a pinch in the lower back

INFORMATION

NUMBER OF REPETITIONS 2–3 sets.

CAUTIONS For back and shoulder problems, omit this exercise. For knee problems, proceed with caution— either omit it or keep the range of motion smaller.

VISUALIZATION As you lift, imagine you have pushed up from the seabed and are breaking the surface of the water to see the light.

PRECISION POINTS

- The pelvis and hips stay pressed into the mat as the heels kick.

- The legs are so strong in the centerline connection that they cannot be parted.
- The legs must stay on the mat as you lift the upper body.
- As you lift, the neck is lengthened and the eyes look at the horizon, with the chest opened.
- The head is only turned after the count of 3, and before it touches the mat.
- There is a dynamic rhythm, with three beats to the kick and the beats to the lift.

Neck Pull

GOALS: ✓ Strengthens the abdominals, in shortened and
lengthened positions

✓ Brings flexibility to the spine and hamstrings

✓ Promotes articulation of the spine

1 Lie on your back with your hands behind your head, one hand cupping the back of your skull and the other supporting it lower on the neck; they

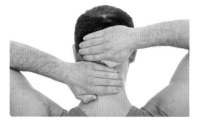

work together to keep the back of your neck lengthened, not to put pressure on the neck. Your feet should be hip-width apart and flexed, so that your toes are pulled up strongly toward your nose, with your powerhouse hollowing your stomach. Your legs should be active—with the energy reaching away through your heels opposing the energy from the powerhouse lengthening your trunk—and with your spine imprinted on the mat.

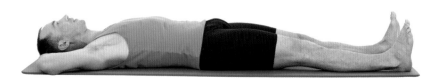

2 **Inhale and initiate rolling up, with your chin to your chest; lift your ribs up over your abdomen, with your powerhouse pulled in deeply to create a C-curve.** Your legs should be sunk into the mat, reaching your heels out in front of you. Your elbows should stay wide. Exhale and deepen the C-curve as your lifted spine takes your upper body over your legs.

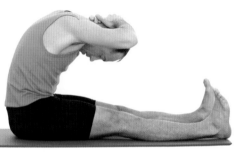

3 **Inhale to unroll your spine from its base and sit tall out of your hips.** Pinch your seat and hinge back from your hips with a lengthened spine.

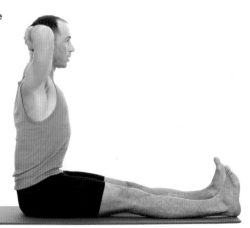

4 **Exhale, tucking your tailbone under toward your heels,** and roll your spine to the mat, placing each vertebra down one at a time, creating a space between them.

> **TRANSITION** Lie flat on your back, with your arms by your side and legs at a 90° angle to the ceiling, ready for Scissors (Shoulder Stand).

MODIFICATIONS

If you have difficulty articulating your spine due to stiffness or weak abdominals, use a slight bend in the knees as you roll up; use your hands to walk up your thighs and, as you bend forward, straighten your legs, then bend your knees again slightly as you prepare to roll the spine back down.

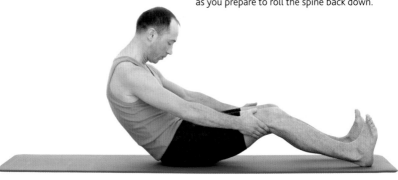

COMMON ERRORS

- The legs lifting as you roll up and down
- The elbows collapsing in, pulling on the neck with the hands, and the chin poking forward
- Using momentum to get off the mat

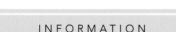

INFORMATION

NUMBER OF REPETITIONS 3–5.

CAUTIONS For back and neck issues, proceed with caution; if in doubt, omit this exercise—it requires a lot of strength and control to do it correctly. If you have difficulties with articulating the spine, use the Modifications.

VISUALIZATION Your legs feel like thay are cemented into the mat; they cannot move.

PRECISION POINTS

- Reaching through the heels toward the opposite wall keeps the legs on the mat.
- Even though the legs are hip-width apart, the centerline is kept strong and the seat is kept active.
- The elbows stay wide; reach them to opposite walls.
- Both of the sides of the trunk stay lengthened.

Scissors (Shoulder Stand)

GOALS: ✓ Opens the hips to stretch the quads and hip flexors

✓ Trains strength of the powerhouse in an inverted position

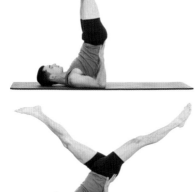

1 **Lie on your back with your legs at at a 90° angle to the ceiling.** Your arms should be long by your side, and your shoulders down your back; lengthen your neck through the crown of your head.

2 **In one smooth movement, press your legs and hips toward the ceiling and place your hands on your lower back, with your elbows in line with your shoulders.** Use the lift of your hips and powerhouse to keep you from sinking into your lower back and onto your hands.

3 **Inhale and, with your abdominals and buttocks engaged,** reach your right leg long toward the mat, and scissor your left leg over your head.

4 Exhale and scissor your legs to change position, reaching away in opposition, with your legs in a split position in the air. If you can remain stable, double-pulse the legs as you reach them away.

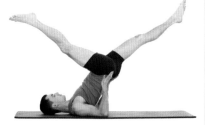

TRANSITION Remain with your legs in the air and your hands supporting your back, ready for Bicycles (Shoulder Stand).

COMMON ERRORS

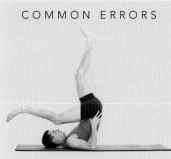

- The legs falling out of the frame
- Sinking into the lower back
- Letting gravity take the weight of the legs, which then fall too far over the head
- Letting the weight fall into the neck—keep it lifted
- The pelvis shifting as the legs move

INFORMATION

NUMBER OF REPETITIONS
3 on each leg.

CAUTIONS For back, neck, shoulder or wrist problems, omit this exercise. If you have difficulty weight-bearing on your shoulders, wrists and elbows, proceed with caution.

VISUALIZATION The legs move like the blades of a pair of scissors.

PRECISION POINTS
- The legs stay long—don't let the knees go soggy and bend.
- The frame is held, and the legs scissor along the centerline.
- The hips and powerhouse are kept lifted throughout.
- The emphasis is on the leg reaching to the mat.

Bicycles (Shoulder Stand)

GOALS:
✓ Opens the hips to stretch the quads and hip flexors
✓ Trains the strength of the powerhouse in an inverted position
✓ Improves coordination of the legs, which in turn further challenges your stability

1 Lie on your back, with your legs and hips toward the ceiling, supported by your hands on your lower back, and your elbows in line with your shoulders. Your legs should be in the Pilates stance, reaching long toward the ceiling. You may need to adjust your hand position, to help support the hips.

2 **Breathing naturally, lengthen your right leg to the mat,** then move your left leg to the ceiling then over your head.

As the right leg reaches away, bend your knee and bring the heel into toward your right buttock, as your left leg reaches long.

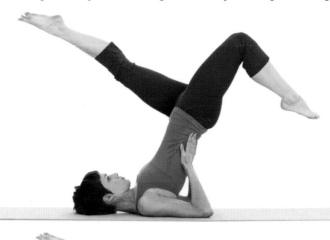

3 Begin to draw your right knee in to your chest.

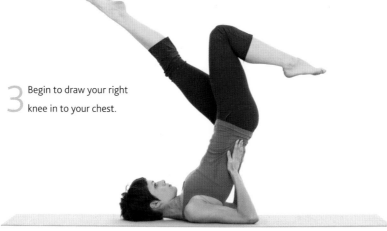

4 **Continue to draw the right knee in further,** and move your left leg straight toward the ceiling again.

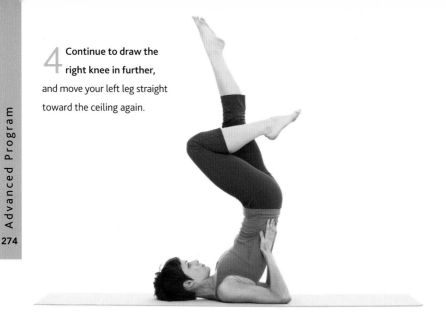

5 **Lengthen your left leg to the mat and complete the bicycling motion** **with the opposite leg.** Pedal smoothly for 3 repetitions, then reverse to pedal backward.

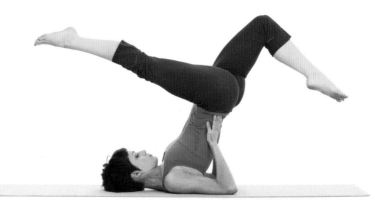

TRANSITION Bend both knees into your chest and roll your spine to the mat with control, ready for the Shoulder Bridge. For a more advanced and challenging transition, keep both hands on your lower back and then lower both feet to the mat; adjust your hands so that the heels of your hands are under your hips, and your fingers are wrapped around the front of your body.

MODIFICATIONS

None. This is a very challenging move, so omit it if necessary and focus instead on the Shoulder Bridge Preparation on page 172.

COMMON ERRORS

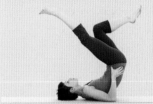

- Sinking into the lower back
- Losing control of the motion of the legs, with the lower back arching
- Letting the weight fall into the neck—keep it lifted.
- The pelvis and trunk shifting or rotating as the legs move

INFORMATION

NUMBER OF REPETITIONS
3 sets in each direction.

CAUTIONS For back, neck, shoulder or wrist problems, omit this exercise. If you have difficulty bearing weight on your shoulders, wrists and elbows, proceed with caution.

VISUALIZATION Imagine you are pedalling through molasses.

PRECISION POINTS
- The bicycling motion should be smooth, slow and precise, with the biggest circles you can make.
- The emphasis is on the leg reaching to the mat; take it as low as possible to open the hip, then draw the heel into the seat. Draw the powerhouse in, to keep the spine lifted and the trunk stable, as the legs move.

Shoulder Bridge

GOALS: ✓ Trains control and stability of the pelvis and lower trunk

✓ Strengthens the powerhouse, buttocks and hamstrings

✓ Opens up the hips and lengthens the hip flexors

✓ Challenges the powerhouse to work in a different position, and when lengthened

1 **Lie on the mat with your knees bent,** hip-width apart, and legs parallel.

2 **Press your hips toward the ceiling, with a squeeze of your buttocks to make a bridge position;** cup your hands under your hips, with your thumbs and fingers wrapped round the front; your elbows should be drawn in and under your hands.

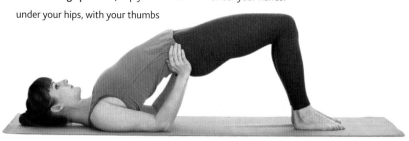

3 **Extend the right leg off the mat, with your thighs still parallel;** your pelvis should remain level, as you create a long line from the toe to the shoulder.

4 **Inhale and kick your right leg to the ceiling;** aim for the leg to be perpendicular to the floor, without losing your alignment.

5 **Flex your foot, exhale and reach your right leg long out of the hip,** until it is level with the left leg.

6 **If you can keep the pelvis and trunk stable,** you can progress by lowering your right leg further, parallel to the mat as you reach it longer. Kick up 3 times, then change legs.

TRANSITION Remove your hands from under your hips and roll down your spine onto the mat. Lengthen your legs and come up to a sitting position, ready for Spine Twist.

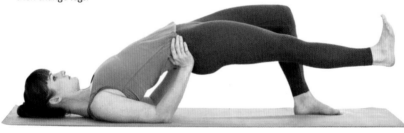

MODIFICATIONS

If your wrists or elbows are not robust enough to weight-bear, leave your arms alongside your body on the mat, as for the intermediate variation, Shoulder Bridge

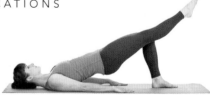

Preparation, on page 172. Keep your pelvis square, and maintain the box. If your spine is not happy to extend high enough to rest your hips on your hands, use the Modification opposite.

COMMON ERRORS

- Losing the box and centerline
- Losing the connection of the powerhouse and ribs when the hips are lifted up
- Losing the level line of the hips when lifting a leg
- The chest and neck sinking, causing strain on the neck

INFORMATION

NUMBER OF REPETITIONS
3 lifts on each leg.

CAUTIONS For back, neck, shoulder or wrist problems, omit this exercise or use the intermediate version on page 172. If you have difficulty weight-bearing on your shoulders, wrists and elbows, proceed with caution and use the intermediate version on page 172.

VISUALIZATION A helium balloon tied to the hips keeps them elevated, as you lengthen your leg. Your leg sweeps long and strong, like a windscreen wiper.

PRECISION POINTS
- The shoulders stay open and the neck remains long.
- Movement is along your centerline; keep the box.
- The powerhouse and ribs stay engaged.
- The pelvis remains level when lifting the leg.
- The powerhouse anchors the pelvis, as the leg moves freely.
- There is a dynamic, kick-up with energy, but with control; lengthen long out of the hip.

Spine Twist

GOALS: ✓ Trains the powerhouse to lift the spine against gravity

                ✓ Brings flexibility to the hamstrings

                ✓ Improves rotation of the spine

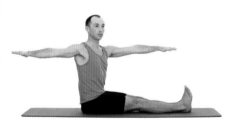

1 **Sit in the middle of the mat, with your legs extended and pressed together,** your feet flexed and your arms reaching in opposite directions—but with your hands in the periphery of your vision. Grow tall on your sit-bones, lifting out of your hips.

2 **Inhale, grow taller out of the hips and, as you exhale to twist to the right, twist again.** Your pelvis should remain rooted on the mat, and your arms stay in line with your shoulders.

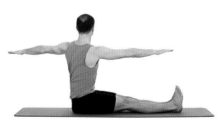

3 **Inhale and return to the center, growing taller through the crown of your head,** with your legs pressed together and your backside working. Exhale and twist twice to the left.

> **TRANSITION** Roll down onto the mat and lift your legs to the ceiling, with your arms by your sides, ready for Jackknife.

MODIFICATIONS

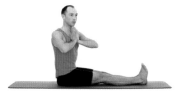

For shoulder problems, exclude the arms by bringing your hands together in a prayer position, and keep your nose in line with your hands. **For tight hamstrings or a tight lower back**, sit on a block to gain the lift out of your hips.

COMMON ERRORS

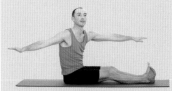

- Slumping back on the hip bones in the sitting position
- The arms swinging around, rather than moving as one with the body
- The legs sliding forward relative to one another
- The shoulders sliding toward the ears

INFORMATION

NUMBER OF REPETITIONS

3 each way.

CAUTIONS For shoulder problems, use the Modifications. For minor back injuries and difficulties with flexibility, proceed with caution. For acute back injuries or disc problems, omit this exercise.

VISUALIZATION Wring the air out of your lungs, like squeezing water from a sponge.

PRECISION POINTS

- Twisting comes from the waist, not from the arms.
- The spine stays lifted and lengthened.
- The arms and shoulders stay in one long line; the arms are carried round in the twist by the movement of the body.
- The eyes look behind you, as you twist to deepen the stretch.
- Pressure is directed out through the heels—reach them toward the wall in front of you.

Jackknife

GOALS: ✓ Brings flexibility to the muscles of the spine

✓ Trains reverse articulation of the spine

✓ Trains strength in the powerhouse, by using it to lower
   the body down from an inverted position

✓ Builds strength in the hips

1 **Lie on your back with your legs
toward the ceiling in the Pilates
stance,** your arms reaching long by your
side and your spine lengthened from
crown to tail.

2 Inhale and lift your hips, by squeezing your powerhouse, to jackknife your legs overhead, aiming to get your feet over your eyes, and your legs on the diagonal.

3 Push your legs further over your head, but going no lower than parallel with the mat. Your arms should stay pressed into the mat, with your neck remaining lengthened.

4 Squeeze your buttocks more, to lift your hips over your shoulders, extending your legs long and strong toward the ceiling, with your fingers reaching in front of you.

5 Exhale and, using your powerhouse, lower your spine onto the mat, vertebra by vertebra; feel the opposition as your feet reach toward the ceiling and your powerhouse controls your descent, until your tailbone lands gently on the mat, and your legs are at a 90° angle again. Inhale to lift your legs again.

To progress this exercise, omit taking the legs overhead parallel to the floor; instead snap them straight toward the ceiling in one strong, long line. When your tailbone lowers to the mat and your legs reach a 90° angle, reach them away further to a 45° angle, before lifting them overhead again.

TRANSITION Lower your legs to the mat and bring your right arm overhead, to roll onto your right side for Side Kick Series: Front/Back.

COMMON ERRORS

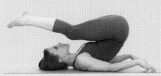

* Throwing the legs overhead and lowering them too far
* Letting the weight fall onto the neck
* Sinking into the neck and spine, rather than lowering with control

INFORMATION

NUMBER OF REPETITIONS 3.

CAUTIONS For back, neck and shoulder problems, omit this exercise.

VISUALIZATION Your legs snap up to the ceiling as if released by a spring. As you lower down, imagine that you are pushing your heels into someone's cupped hands, to keep your hips forward.

PRECISION POINTS

* The arms work with energy throughout, and stay lengthened, with the fingers reaching forward.
* The weight goes onto the shoulders, not the neck.
* The powerhouse and hips are used to generate the movement.
* The legs are active in a Pilates stance.
* When the legs are toward the ceiling, a long line is created through the trunk, hips and knees.
* The feet stay over the eyes as you lower down.

Side Kick Series: Front/Back

GOALS:
✓ Tones, lengthens and strengthens the legs, hips and abdominals

✓ Creates length in the hamstrings

✓ Challenges stability and balance further, as the movement of the leg progresses in the advanced exercise

1 **Lie on your side, in line with the back edge of the mat.** Support yourself on your elbow, and take that hand to the back of your head to support it and maintain the length in the neck. Bring your top hand behind your head and your elbow to the ceiling. Ensure your waist is lifted and lengthened by engaging your powerhouse.

2 **Inhale to lift both legs as one, then bring your feet forward in line with the front corner of the mat and lower your bottom leg.** With your hands behind your head, you will feel less stable than in

the beginner and intermediate Side Kick Series, but will work harder and be challenged more. Be active in your powerhouse, backside and shoulder blade stabilizers and you will be able to maintain your balance while moving your top leg.

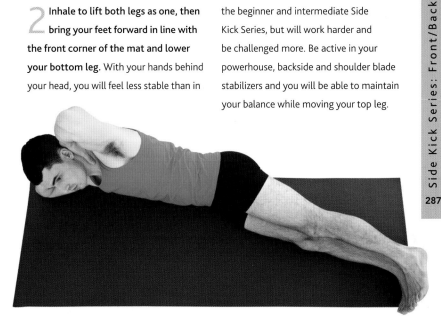

3 **Inhale and, with your top leg at hip-height parallel to the floor,** kick forward with a double pulse: kick-kick.

4 **Sweep your leg back in one long line from your hip toward the back corner of the room;** keep your backside

muscles firm and your knee long. Keep the box as your leg moves through space. Breathe naturally; kick-kick forward, then reach long to kick back.

> **TRANSITION** Stack the top heel on the bottom heel with a slight turn-out, ready for Side Kick Series: Up/Down.

MODIFICATIONS

For neck or shoulder problems, place a block under the head, with the bottom arm extended forward on the mat. Use the right height of block to keep the neck in line with the spine; you may need to experiment

with blocks of different heights, or use more than one. Use the same position when you repeat the exercise on the other side. **For hip replacements,** exercise control and precision. If you need to use either Modification, keep your stabilizing hand on the mat.

COMMON ERRORS

- The hips and shoulders rocking and rolling
- The top elbow moving in space
- The top leg swinging around without control
- Losing the long line of the spine, causing it to bend and extend with the movement of the leg

INFORMATION

NUMBER OF REPETITIONS 5–10.

CAUTIONS If you have hips that clunk or have had hip replacements, work in a restricted range of movement, with the seat muscles active. For neck and shoulder problems, follow the Modifications.

VISUALIZATION The top leg swings like a pendulum on a clock.

PRECISION POINTS
- Keep the spine long, from the top of the head to the tip of the tailbone, as the leg moves.
- The focus of the eyes is on the wall in front.
- The top hip and shoulder stay directed to the ceiling.
- The moving leg is lengthened and active, with no buckle in the knee.
- Top elbow always stays pointing to the ceiling.

Side Kick Series: Up/Down

GOALS: ✓ Tones, lengthens and strengthens the legs, hips and abdominals

✓ Challenges the length of the adductor muscles of the inner thigh

✓ Trains stability and balance in the side-lying position

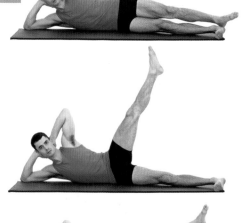

1 **Lie in your side-lying position, with your top hand behind your head and the elbow to the ceiling.** Your top heel should be in contact with your bottom heel, with the top leg slightly turned out.

2 **Inhale and lift your top leg straight up,** keeping the top hip in line over the bottom hip.

3 **To lower the leg,** exhale and resist your own movement as you reach the leg long.

TRANSITION Return to the
starting position for Passé.

Side Kick Series: Up/Down

291

MODIFICATIONS

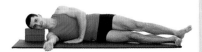

For neck and shoulder problems,
use a block under the head at the
correct height. **For hip problems
and hip replacements,** keep the
lift of the leg smaller.

COMMON ERRORS

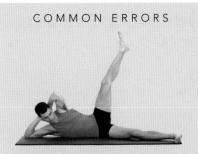

- Losing the stack of the hips as the leg lifts
- The shoulder blades not staying connected
  to the back and lifting to the ears
- The powerhouse switching off, allowing the
  waist to collapse onto the mat
- Losing the energy in the top leg so that the
  knee bends and turns in

INFORMATION

NUMBER OF REPETITIONS 5.

CAUTIONS For hip problems,
including hip replacements and hips
that clunk, keep the movement smaller
and work with active seat muscles. For
neck and shoulder problems, follow the
Modification.

VISUALIZATION Lift up a 1-ton
weight; pull down a 2-ton weight.

PRECISION POINTS
- Maintain the box, with the hips and
  shoulders vertically aligned.
- Reach through the crown of the
  head, with the eyes facing forward.
- The top elbow stays pointing to the
  ceiling, with the chest open.
- Maintain stability in the trunk as
  the leg moves.
- Keep the scoop, with the waist lifted.

Side Kick Series: Passé

GOALS:
✓ Challenges and trains balance with the movement of the leg
✓ Tones, lengthens and strengthens the abdominals, buttocks and thighs
✓ Challenges the flexibility of the hips

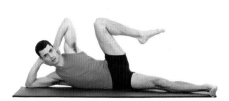

1 **Lie on your side, with your top hand behind your head, elbow to the ceiling.** Line your top leg on top of your bottom leg, with both heels together and the top knee slightly turned to the ceiling. With the big toe of your top leg, trace the inside of the bottom leg to the knee.

2 **Breathing naturally, lift your knee toward your top ear;** open your hip and keep the pelvis square.

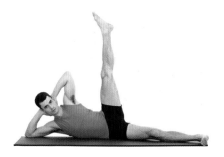

3 **Lengthen your leg to the ceiling, with a turn-out to open the hip.** Reach the leg long out of your hip to lower it to hip height. Repeat 3 times; then reverse, by kicking the leg up first toward the shoulder; bend the knee and lengthen the leg, sliding your big toe along your lower leg.

MODIFICATIONS

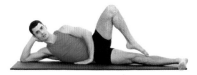

For stiff hips or hip problems, reduce the range by sliding your big toe along the lower leg; omit the lift to the ceiling. **If you are struggling with balance,** use your top hand to stabilize you, by placing it on the mat in front of you. **If you have neck or shoulder problems,** use a block of the right height under your head, with the lower arm extended.

COMMON ERRORS

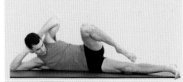

- Not keeping the hips stacked
- The chest rolling forward and the elbow of the top arm moving around in space, rolling forward or falling backward
- Losing the length of the spine, with the eyes on the feet
- The waist sinking into the mat

INFORMATION

NUMBER OF REPETITIONS
3 each way on each leg.

CAUTIONS For hip problems or 'clunking' hips, reduce the range; follow the Modifications, keeping the seat wrapped, and aim to progress gradually to the bigger movement as you improve.

VISUALIZATION Move to a beat of 4 points—slide, lift, straighten, lower—then smooth the corners to create a sense of flow.

PRECISION POINTS
- Keep the waist lifted throughout.
- The spine stays lengthened, reaching through the crown of the head, with the eyes forward.
- The top elbow stays static in space, pointing to the ceiling.

Side Kick Series: Circles

GOALS: ✓ Challenges stability in the pelvis and trunk

✓ Tones, lengthens and strengthens the abdominals, buttocks and thighs

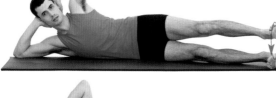

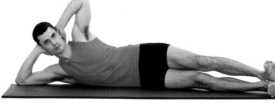

TRANSITION Bend your top leg and place the foot flat on the mat in front of you. Hold the ankle with your top hand and work the knee toward the ceiling, ready for Inner Thigh Lifts and Circles.

1 **Lie in your side-lying position, with your top hand behind your head and the elbow to the ceiling.** Your top leg should at hip height, reaching away.

2 **Breathing naturally, create small dynamic circles, with the instep of your top foot brushing the heel of your bottom foot.** After 5–8 repetitions maintain your leg at hip height and reverse the circles.

MODIFICATIONS

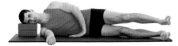

For neck and shoulder problems, use a block under your head to take the strain off your neck. **If you struggle to keep your hips stacked and maintain balance,** place your top hand on the mat in front of you, with your bottom arm straight out in front of you.

COMMON ERRORS

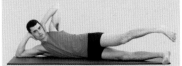

- Moving the leg from the foot, rather than the hip
- The powerhouse switching off, so that the abdominals fall forward onto the mat
- Not stabilizing, so that the hips roll around
- Fixing the eyes on the feet, rather than in front, causing the spine to bend
- The elbow of the top arm moving around in space

INFORMATION

NUMBER OF REPETITIONS 5–8.

CAUTIONS For neck and shoulder problems, follow the Modifications.

VISUALIZATION Circle the top leg around the inside of a power circle.

PRECISION POINTS
- The top leg stays at hip height, lengthened but loose, without tensing the thigh muscles.
- Move from the hip, not the knee or ankle.
- The pelvis stays stable, with an active powerhouse and seat muscles.
- The top elbow stays still, pointing to the ceiling.

Side Kick Series:
Inner Thigh Lifts and Circles

GOALS: ✓ Creates muscle balance by working the inner thighs

✓ Stretches out the hip and buttock of the leg that has just worked

1 **Lie in your side-lying position.** Bend your top leg and place the foot flat on the floor in front of you, with the knee toward the ceiling, holding the ankle with

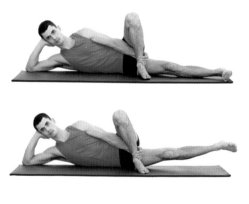

your top hand. Use your powerhouse to keep your trunk lengthened and active as you bend the top leg; the top foot should feel firmly planted into the mat. Then work the top knee toward the ceiling to create a perpendicular angle; you will have to keep the hip active to maintain that angle.

2 **Breathe naturally and lengthen the lower leg to lift it; keep the knee facing forward.** Lengthen the leg longer out of the hip, to lower it to hover just above the mat. You can pulse the lift, to challenge the inside of the thigh muscles.

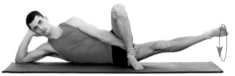

3 **On completing the last lift, the leg stays at hip height to make circles from the hip:** forward 5–8 times, then reverse.

TRANSITION Slide the top leg over the lower leg, to set up for Hot Potato.

MODIFICATIONS

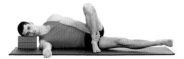

For neck or shoulder problem that prevent you resting your head on your hand, place your head on a block at the right height, to keep your neck in line with the rest of your spine. **If you have a knee problem,** rest the top knee on the floor.

COMMON ERRORS

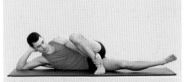

* The working leg losing energy, letting the knee bend and the ankle go floppy
* Lifting the leg from the foot that is turned in, rather than lifting cleanly from the inner thigh
* Losing the box, so that the top hip rolls forward or back

INFORMATION

NUMBER OF REPETITIONS 5–8.

CAUTIONS For stiff hips and knees, don't hold the ankle; if necessary, follow the Modifications. For neck issues, use the modified beginner's version on page 124.

VISUALIZATION Balance a champagne glass on the inside of your knee; don't lose a drop!

PRECISION POINTS
* Maintain the box, with the eyes on a point in front of you.
* The working leg is long and strong throughout.
* Lift from the inner thigh muscles and the hip, not the foot.

Side Kick Series: Hot Potato

GOALS: ✓ Tones the buttocks, thighs and abdominals

✓ Teaches the ability to stabilize the trunk while generating large destabilizing movements in the leg

✓ Cultivates flexibility of the hip joints

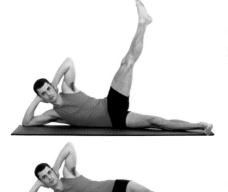

1 Set yourself up in your side-lying position along the back edge of the mat, as you did for the beginning of Side Kick Series; place your top hand behind your head, with the shoulder blade engaged down your back. Tap the heel of your top foot behind your lower foot 4 times.

2 Kick your top leg to the ceiling, in line with your hip.

3 Lower your upper foot in front of your lower foot and tap the heel 4 times; kick up, lower behind and tap the heel 3 times. Kick up again, lower in front and tap the heel again 3 times. Repeat with a diminishing number of heel taps, with kicks in between; then kick up once in each direction.

TRANSITION Return to your starting position ready for Grande Ronde de Jambe.

MODIFICATIONS

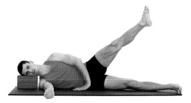

For a stiff neck, use a block under your head, and bring your bottom arm through in line with your shoulder. Ensure your head, neck and spine are aligned.

COMMON ERRORS

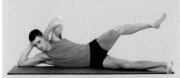

- The kicking leg wavering around with a bent knee—keep it long and strong
- The hips rolling forward and back
- The back arching and bending as the leg moves
- Sinking into the waist and shoulders

INFORMATION

NUMBER OF REPETITIONS

4 sets of heel taps and kicks.

CAUTIONS For hip pain, omit this exercise. If you have very mobile hips that click or clunk, keep the range of movement smaller and ensure that you work your deep hip muscles; when you have greater stability you will be able to aim for the full range of movement.

VISUALIZATION You have a spring attached to your top foot; you resist the spring to tap the heel, and control the recoil to kick up.

PRECISION POINTS

- The hips stay stacked, with the upper one on top of the lower one in one neat line.
- The waist stays lifted and active.
- The hip is turned out as you lift the leg.
- Length is created in the leg and trunk by reaching out of the hip; your powerhouse reaches through the crown of your head, as the leg reaches long in the opposite direction.
- The top leg stays lengthened.

Side Kick Series: Grande Ronde de Jambe

GOALS: ✓ Brings flexibility to the hip joint, hamstrings and hip flexors

✓ Tones the buttocks, thighs and abdominals

✓ Teaches how to stabilize the trunk, while encountering large destabilizing movements in the leg

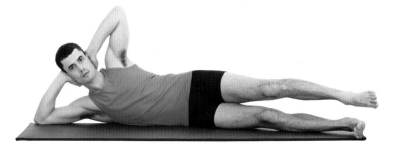

1 **In your side-lying position,** move your legs forward to 45° in a Pilates stance and your top hand behind your head.

2 **Breathing naturally,** take your leg to the front, parallel to the floor.

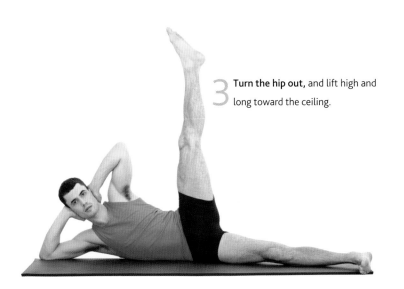

3 **Turn the hip out,** and lift high and long toward the ceiling.

4 **Press your hip forward as you lengthen the leg back behind the hip, to make the biggest circle in the air that you can with your foot.** Then the leg continues forward as it brushes the lower leg to circle again, for 3 repetitions. Then reverse the circle, by taking the leg back behind the hip.

TRANSITION Return to the starting position and bring your top leg out in front, in line with the hip and parallel to the floor, ready for Bicycle.

MODIFICATIONS

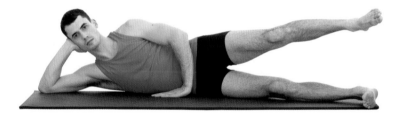

If you have difficulty in preventing yourself wobbling, bring your top hand to the mat to use it as a stabilizer.
For problems with flexibility or hip pain, keep the circles smaller.

COMMON ERRORS

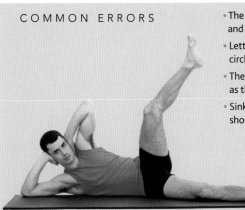

- The hips rolling forward and back
- Letting the knee on the circling leg bend
- The back arching and bending, as the leg moves
- Sinking into the waist and the shoulders

INFORMATION

NUMBER OF REPETITIONS

3 each way and on each leg.

CAUTIONS For hip pain, omit this exercise. If you have very mobile hips that click or clunk, keep the range smaller and ensure that you work your deep hip muscles; when you have greater stability, you will gradually be able to make bigger circles without any clicking or clunking in the hip.

VISUALIZATION Your foot lightly traces the outside of a very large hoop.

PRECISION POINTS

- The hips stay stacked, with the upper hip on top of the lower one, in one neat line.
- The waist stays lifted and active.
- The hip is turned out as you go to lift the leg.
- The top leg stays long and strong throughout the circle.
- Length is created in the leg and trunk by reaching out of the hip; your powerhouse reaches through the crown of the head, as the leg reaches long in the opposite direction.

Side Kick Series: Bicycle

GOALS:
✓ Challenges core stability
✓ Strengthens the hip and leg
✓ Opens the front of the hip

1 **In your side-lying position,** move your legs forward to a 45° angle in a Pilates stance and your top hand behind your head.

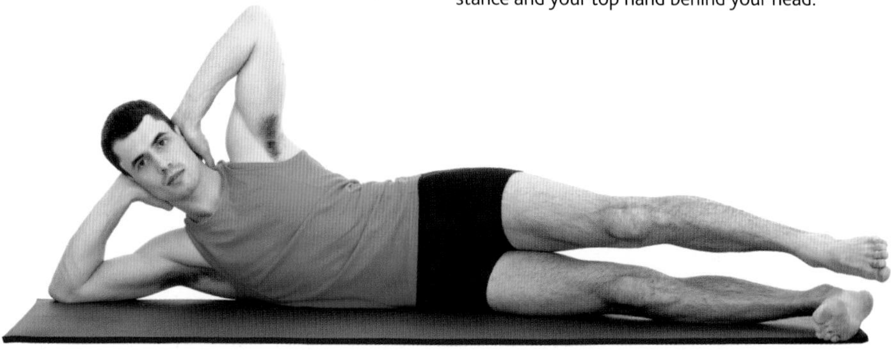

2 **Sweep the top leg forward as far in front as you can,** level with your hip and parallel to the floor.

3 **Bend the knee to your chest,** and work the heel toward your seat.

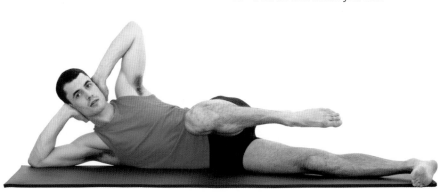

4 **Brush the lower thigh with your top thigh, as you take the bent leg back as far as you can, keeping your spine long.** Extend the leg back behind you, and finish

the bicycle motion by sweeping the leg forward as far as it will go. Repeat 3 times; then reverse the pedalling motion, taking the straight leg back, bringing the heel to your seat with the top hip pressed forward, bringing the knee to your chest, then straightening the leg to repeat it.

TRANSITION Lift your lower leg to your top leg, pull in your abdominals and roll onto your belly, with your forehead on your hands, for Beats on the Belly (see page 190) as the transition to repeating this series on the other side. After completing both sides, roll onto your back, with your arms by your sides and your legs toward the ceiling, for Teaser I.

MODIFICATIONS

If you feel really unstable, work with your top hand on the mat until you can balance well enough to complete the bicycling motion without wobbling off your hip.
For neck problems, rest your head on a block, or on your outstretched arm, in a position where your neck doesn't feels any strain. Keep the range smaller until you have the stamina to complete 3 repetitions each way, cleanly.

COMMON ERRORS

- The top leg dropping toward the mat
- The trunk and pelvis rolling around as the leg moves
- The top leg rolling in

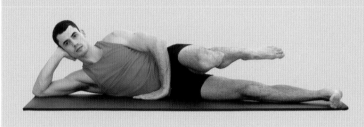

INFORMATION

NUMBER OF REPETITIONS
3 each way, on each leg.

CAUTIONS For hip pain, proceed with caution; either keep the movements much smaller or omit this exercise. It is quite common to feel a degree of effort and tiredness in the hip and thigh muscles on completing the whole of the Side Kick Series; don't be discouraged—this isn't pain, just muscle fatigue.

VISUALIZATION You are riding a bicycle with huge wheels in a high gear; you have to press hard through the pedals and reach your legs long.

PRECISION POINTS
- The hips and shoulders stay stacked.
- The leg goes back behind the hip, and the hip is pressed forward, as you bicycle.
- The waist is kept lifted and the body is stable throughout.
- The leg reaches long out of the hip.

Teaser I

1 **Lie on your back, scoop your powerhouse, bend both knees into the chest and lengthen your legs out to 45° in the Pilates stance.** Your arms should be over your head on the mat, with your neck and sides lengthened. Your powerhouse is very active, with your legs wrapped from the rear and your ribs flush with your front as your arms reach behind you.

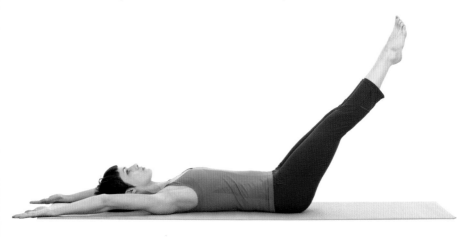

2 **Inhale to prepare; exhale as you lift your arms and peel your head and spine off the mat, bone by bone,** to reach your fingers toward your toes, floating up as if your upper body weighs nothing.

3 **Pause and "tease" to find the balance, back a little on your tailbone,** with your abdominals holding the C-curve and your chest lifted toward the sky.

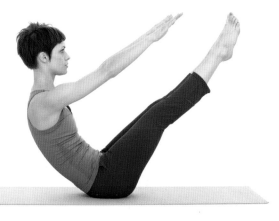

4 Inhale and tuck your tailbone under more, to roll your body away with control, with your legs staying static in space. Create length as you reach the mat, with your arms overhead as in the starting position. Exhale and roll up.

TRANSITION Being mindful of your signs of readiness for the Teaser series: if you are ready for Teaser II, then remain in your balance position. If you are not ready for the remainder of the Teaser series, bend your knees and place your feet on the mat with 'tippy toes' for Cancan.

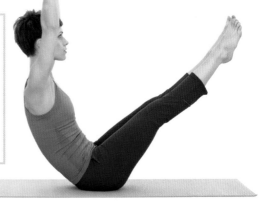

MODIFICATIONS

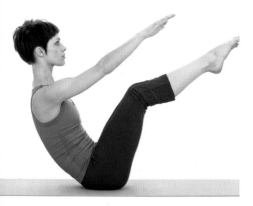

To build up to Teaser I, particularly for those with weak abdominals, those who are deconditioned and for tight hamstrings: soften your knees, so that they bend the minimum amount to enable you to hold the balance with the C-curve, and without your abdominals bulging. Roll back, roll up, lengthen your legs as far as you can, soften the knees and roll back again. If you need a little more support, place your hands lightly behind the thighs.

COMMON ERRORS

- Losing control of the legs, so that they lower to the floor as you roll up and down
- The abdominals bulging, and the back arching
- Throwing the upper body up by the shoulders to come back up, rather than rolling the spine sequentially
- Working from the shoulders, head and neck, rather than the abdominals, to roll up.

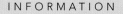

INFORMATION

NUMBER OF REPETITIONS 3.

CAUTIONS For lower back issues, follow the Pilates principles (see pages 24–7) when doing this exercise and be very mindful of your own ability. Use the Modification that represents the correct level for you. For a stiff lower back, follow the modified Teaser I Leg on page 194.

VISUALIZATION An invisible force pulls your fingers to your toes, as you roll up to find your balance. Your spine rolls like a wheel.

PRECISION POINTS

- The legs stay still in the same point in space; they don't lower or wobble around.
- The inner thighs and buttocks are kept working throughout.
- The powerhouse is strongly engaged throughout.
- The spine moves with precision and control, bone by bone.
- The breath flows with the exercise, rather than being held.
- The ribs stay engaged when reaching the arms over the head.

Teaser II

GOALS: ✓ Strengthens the lower abdominals

✓ Challenges you to maintain balance and work with control

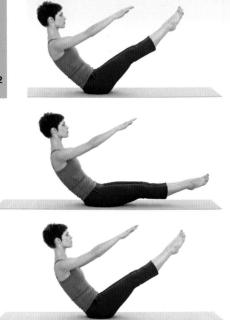

1 **After lying on your back, scoop your powerhouse, bend both knees into the chest and lengthen your legs out to 45° in the Pilates stance.** Rest in a balance on your tailbone, with your scoop holding you there, a C-curve in your lower back, your arms parallel with your legs, and your fingers reaching toward your toes, in a V-position.

2 **Inhale and, keeping your body perfectly still,** lower your legs toward the mat.

3 **Exhale and swiftly lift your legs back to the V-position.** Repeat for 3 lowers and lifts.

TRANSITION if you can maintain the slight C-curve without your lower back buckling, and keep the balance in Teaser II, then you are ready for Teaser III. If your stamina is not robust enough to continue, bend your knees and place your tiptoes on the mat, ready for Cancan.

MODIFICATIONS

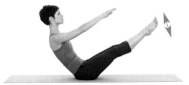

If necessary, keep the range of motion of your legs smaller, until you are strong enough to lower them to the mat and return. **If you have tight hamstrings,** slightly soften your knees, but keep your feet above your knees.

COMMON ERRORS

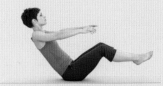

- Tipping the head back as the legs lower
- Losing control of the powerhouse as the legs lower and lift, so that the abdominals bulge and the back arches
- The body lowering, as the legs lower to the floor
- Losing the centerline connection in the legs, and the legs falling apart

INFORMATION

NUMBER OF REPETITIONS 3.

CAUTIONS For lower back problems, omit this exercise. If you have a tender tailbone, proceed with caution.

VISUALIZATION Your abdominals are a tight coil; you carefully gain spaces between the coils as you lower your legs, and the recoil brings your legs back up.

PRECISION POINTS

- Keep the lower back and chest lifted, to create length in the back of the neck.
- The eyes are on the horizon.
- The arms are parallel with the legs, with the shoulder blades engaged down the back.
- The legs are zipped up together in the centerline, in the Pilates stance.
- The backs of the legs are wrapped.
- Movement is executed with control.

Teaser III

GOALS: ✓ Trains stamina and strength in the abdominals

✓ Poses a huge challenge to control

✓ Brings the components of Teaser I and Teaser II together,
to work the upper and lower portions of the abdominals

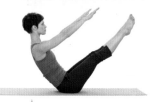

1 **Balance your legs and spine in a V-position,** with your arms parallel with your legs.

2 **Lift your arms,** so that they are parallel to your ears.

3 **Exhale and initiate the roll-down,** by scooping deeper into your spine and lowering one vertebra at a time onto the mat, with your upper body and legs lengthening away simultaneously.

4 **Your arms and legs lower until they hover just above the mat, reaching away from a very strong center.** Inhale and spring back to the V-position, with your arms and legs coming up simultaneously; reach toward your toes and balance. Lift your arms alongside your ears to roll down again.

TRANSITION Bend your knees and place the tips of your toes on the mat; put your hands on the mat behind your hips, ready for Cancan.

MODIFICATIONS

If you do not have the strength or stamina in your abdominals to execute Teaser III accurately, use the right level of Teaser 1 Leg (see page 192), or Teaser I (see page 196) or II (see page 312), for you. Build up your stamina and strength gradually, until you are able to do Teaser III safely.

COMMON ERRORS

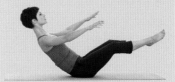

- Losing the scoop, so the back arches
- The legs or body lowering first
- Using momentum rather than control to come back up
- Losing the centerline connection of the legs, and the rib/shoulder blade connection at the shoulders

INFORMATION

NUMBER OF REPETITIONS 3.

CAUTIONS For lower back problems, omit this exercise. If you have a tender tailbone, proceed with caution.

VISUALIZATION Your middle is a strong piece of elastic; it lengthens as the body and legs lower, and springs you back up into the V-position.

PRECISION POINTS

- The arms and legs float up effortlessly.
- The powerhouse lifts and lengthens the spine.
- The wrap of the legs is maintained, with the legs in the Pilates position.
- The scoop is maintained: this move depends on the powerhouse, and without it the wrong muscles will be used.
- The ribs are kept engaged, and the shoulders are sliding down the back.

Cancan

GOALS: ✓ Strengthens the abdominals, particularly the oblique muscles

✓ Teaches how to keep the spine lifted, while the legs move

1 **Sit tall on the mat and place your hands behind your hips, just wider than the mat, with your fingers facing back and your elbows straight.** Bend your knees and place the tips of your toes on the mat; your legs should be drawn tightly into the centerline. Your chest and spine should be lifted.

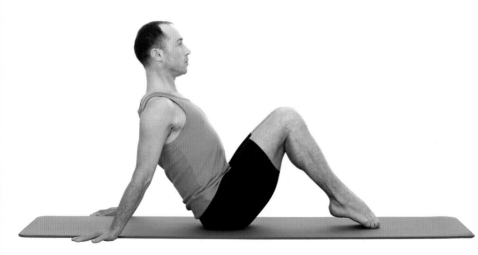

2 **Draw your abdominals in and take your knees to the right;** your toes should stay on the mat in the center, with the lower back lifted.

3 **Take both knees to the left, keeping your chest open and lifted,** your legs pressed together and your toes on tiptoe on the mat.

4 Bring your knees back to the right, then kick both legs up in a strong diagonal, zipped together, with the waist lifted. Bend your knees to return your toes to the mat, then bring your knees to the left to repeat, with a rhythm of 1-2-3-kick, with the kick to alternate sides.

TRANSITION If you can maintain a lifted waist, open chest and long elbows during Cancan, then you are ready for Hip Circles: return your toes to the mat, as for the starting position. To continue your workout omitting Hip Circles, roll down onto your front for Swimming.

MODIFICATIONS

Bend your elbows and bear the weight through your forearms, rather than your hands.

COMMON ERRORS

- The elbows bend when the legs move
- The body twists with the legs
- The chest and lower back sink, with the chin poking forward

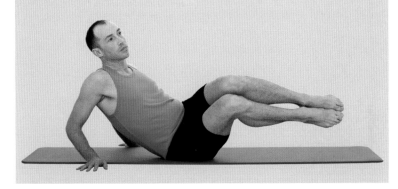

Cancan

319

INFORMATION

NUMBER OF REPETITIONS 3.

CAUTIONS For back problems, omit this exercise. For wrist and elbow problems, follow the Modifications. For shoulder problems, proceed with caution, follow the Modifications or omit the exercise.

VISUALIZATION Kick your legs like a cancan dancer.

PRECISION POINTS

- The elbows stay long, but not locked out.
- The neck, spine and waist stay lifted, with the collarbone open.
- A strong scoop is used throughout.
- The legs are in the Pilates stance, with a wrap of the legs to support the powerhouse.
- The legs kick high.

Hip Circles

GOALS: ✓ Strengthens the abdominals

✓ Teaches the abdominals to stabilize the middle, while the legs move separately

✓ Opens the front of the chest

✓ Creates a huge challenge to stamina, if completed after the Teaser series

1 **Sit tall on the mat and place your hands behind your hips, just wider than the mat, your fingers facing back and your elbows straight.** Bend your knees, and place the tips of your toes on the mat; your legs should be drawn tightly into the centerline. Your chest and spine should be lifted.

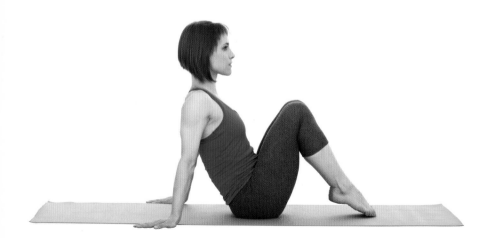

2 Lift your legs into a V-position in the **Pilates stance**. Keep your chest open and your spine lifted.

3 Inhale and take your legs to the right.

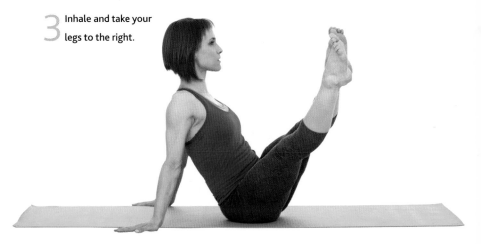

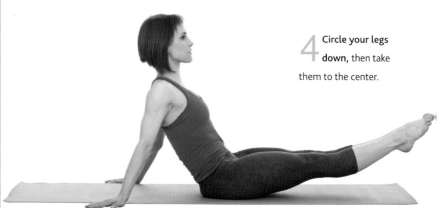

4 **Circle your legs down,** then take them to the center.

5 **Exhale, taking your legs to the left and back up to the center.** Repeat, reversing the circle to the left.

TRANSITION Bend your knees to return your toes to the mat. Then roll down onto your back, take your right arm overhead and roll through your right side onto your front, ready for Swimming.

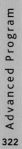

MODIFICATIONS

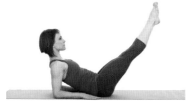

Bend your elbows and weight-bear on your forearms. Begin with smaller circles, and gradually increase the size of the circles as you grow stronger.

COMMON ERRORS

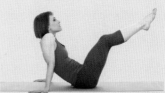

- The chest and lower back sinking, with the chin poking forward
- The elbows bending as the legs move
- The body twisting with the legs
- Losing the centerline and wrap of the legs

INFORMATION

NUMBER OF REPETITIONS

3 sets of circles in each direction.

....

CAUTIONS For back problems, omit this exercise. For wrist and elbow problems, follow the Modification with the elbows bent. For certain shoulder problems, proceed with caution; it may be necessary to omit the exercise.

....

VISUALIZATION You have a pole along the length of your spine that doesn't buckle or bend as you move your legs.

PRECISION POINTS

- The elbows stay long, but not locked out.
- The neck, spine and waist remain lifted, with the collarbone open.
- A strong scoop is used throughout.
- The legs are in the Pilates stance, with a wrap of the legs to support the powerhouse.
- The shoulder blades stay engaged down the back.
- The emphasis is on the up swing of the legs.

Swimming

GOALS: ✓ Trains strength in the spinal muscles

✓ Takes the abdominals into a lengthened position and trains strength at their full length

1 **Lie down on your front, with your forehead on the mat, your arms stretched out in front of you and shoulder-width apart,** your shoulder blades sliding down your back, and your legs pressed together. With your abdominals pulled in, lengthen from the toes to the fingertips.

2 **Inhale and lengthen to lift your right arm,** your left leg and your head level with the right arm, with your powerhouse stabilizing your middle so that you can reach away.

3 **Exhale and, as you lower your right arm and left leg to hover over the mat, lift your other limbs and lengthen from a strong center** . Maintain the lift in all your limbs, with your chest open and your eyes to the horizon. Inhale for a count of 5 as you lift opposing limbs in time with your breath; exhale for a count of 5 as you lift alternating limbs, without them touching the mat.

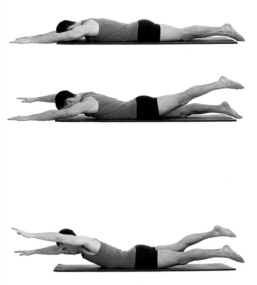

TRANSITION Push back into the Rest Position (see page 170), then lengthen onto your front for Leg Pull Front. Alternatively, lengthen onto your front, hands on the mat under your shoulders, ready for Leg Pull Front.

MODIFICATIONS

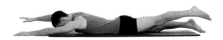

If your lower back pinches with all the limbs lifted, refer to the intermediate version on page 200, and always keep one arm and leg on the mat.

COMMON ERRORS

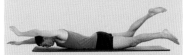

- Losing the centerline connection of the legs, so that they come apart.
- Rotation in the trunk, so that the pelvis and shoulders shift with the lift of the limbs.
- Extending the neck, so that it is strained and not lengthened.
- The shoulders sliding up to the ears, with the elbows bent.

INFORMATION

NUMBER OF REPETITIONS
2 sets of inhale/exhale.

....

CAUTIONS If you have tight shoulders or shoulder problems, limit the lift in the arms or use the modified intermediate version on page 202. For lower back pain or back injuries, proceed with caution; start with the modified intermediate version and keep the lift of the legs low; ensure your scoop is active throughout. Omit this exercise if it is still uncomfortable on the lower back.

VISUALIZATION Lift to swim over the crest of a wave.

....

PRECISION POINTS
- The emphasis is on the lift!
- Reach your limbs away from a strong center, working toward lengthening longer.
- The arms stay in line with the shoulders, with the shoulders down and the back and the elbows lengthened.

Leg Pull Front

GOALS:
- ✓ Strengthens the powerhouse
- ✓ Trains the muscles that stabilize the shoulder blades on the back
- ✓ Challenges the strength of the upper body

1 **Lie on your front, with your palms to the mat under your shoulders,** elbows pressed firmly into your sides, and toes hooked under so that the feet are flexed.

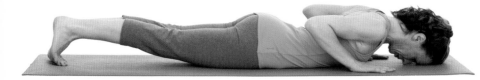

2 **In one move, push up into a plank position,** keeping your legs strongly pressed into the center connection and your abdominals pulled deeply into your spine.

3 **Inhale and lift your right leg to reach behind you, parallel to the floor;** keep the weight equal between both hands, and keep your pelvis square.

4 Exhale and push back on your left heel, so that the **foot flexes and the calf is stretched.** Return the heel over your toes and lower the right foot to the floor. Repeat with the left leg lifted, for a cycle of one inhale and one exhale.

TRANSITION Lower to the floor and sit on the mat, facing forward, for Leg Pull Up. For a more challenging transition, remain in the plank position; bring your right hand to the left, lift your left arm up to the ceiling; your body should follow to face the ceiling as you place your left hand on the mat behind you. With fingers facing forward and heels down—you are now in an inverted plank position.

MODIFICATIONS

To work toward the full move, keep both feet on the mat and push both heels back to the mat simultaneously.

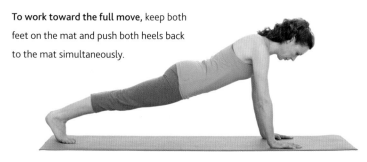

COMMON ERRORS

- Losing the activity in your seat and abdominal muscles, so that the pelvis dips toward the mat and the abdominals sag
- Sinking between the shoulder blades
- The chin poking forward, and the back of the neck straining

INFORMATION

NUMBER OF REPETITIONS

2–3 on each leg.

CAUTIONS For weak wrists and elbows, and for shoulder and back injuries, refer to the intermediate Leg Pull Front Support on page 204 and the Modifications for that level. Foot and ankle problems causing stiffness may provide limitations, and it may not be possible to maintain the Leg Pull Front position: if so, omit this exercise.

VISUALIZATION You are a pole from head to heel; move as one.

PRECISION POINTS

- The heels return over the toes.
- The body is one long line through the ankles, knees, hips, waist, shoulders and neck.
- The shoulders are kept strong, with no "winging" of the shoulder blades.
- The legs are pressed together, like a Greek column.
- The abdominals stay hollowed into the spine to create a clean profile, otherwise they will visibly dip toward the mat.
- The box and frame remain square throughout.

Leg Pull Up

GOALS: ✓ Strengthens the powerhouse, hips and buttocks

✓ Opens the chest and the shoulders

✓ Strengthens the shoulders and upper arms

1 **Sit on the mat, place your hands behind you,** with your fingers facing forward and your legs extended in front of you, wrapped in the Pilates stance.

2 **Inhale and press your hips toward the ceiling,** with your eyes on the horizon, your legs long and strong, and the soles of your feet flat on the mat, creating one long line, in a reverse push-up position.

3 **Exhale and kick one leg up to the ceiling, aiming for the perpendicular, without losing the alignment of the hips and pelvis.** Reach the leg long to lower it, keeping the strong line that you created in the set-up position. Kick the same leg three times in total.

4 Switch legs and kick up for 3 repetitions.

TRANSITION For the advanced transition, keep your hips raised; bend your right knee and slide it underneath you, to kneel on it. Turn your body to the right, with your right hand on the mat under your right shoulder, keeping the left leg at hip height and the left hand behind your head, for the Kneeling Side Kick Series. If your wrists and shoulders are fatigued, simply lower the hips to the mat and kneel, facing the long side of the mat, ready for the Kneeling Side Kick Series.

MODIFICATIONS

Bend the elbows and weight-bear through the forearms. If your wrists and shoulders need to rest when in the full position, lower your hips to the mat when you switch legs.

COMMON ERRORS

- Letting the hips sink as the leg lifts
- Sinking into the shoulders, so that the chin pokes forward and the chest collapses
- The weight-bearing leg rolling out, so that the weight falls on the outside of the foot

INFORMATION

NUMBER OF REPETITIONS

3 on each leg.

CAUTIONS For shoulder issues and carpal-tunnel problems, omit this exercise. With repetitive strain injuries in the wrists, caution is required. For weak or problematic wrists and elbows, use the first Modification. With ankle injuries, caution is required. For a fragile neck, proceed with caution, and omit if necessary.

VISUALIZATION Your body and legs create the third side of a triangle.

PRECISION POINTS

- The eyes are kept on the horizon, with a long neck.
- The elbows stay lengthened, but not locked out.
- The powerhouse and buttocks keep the pelvis pressed up in a line with the body throughout the move.
- The collarbone stay open, with the shoulder blades moving down the back.
- The hands are directly under the shoulders.
- The legs do not bend, but stay long.
- The ribs and abdominals stay engaged and held in.

Kneeling Side Kick Series

GOALS: ✓ Trains dynamic balance

✓ Trains stability in the hips, pelvis and trunk, to tone the muscles of the hips and waist

1 Kneel on the long side of the mat.

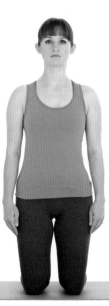

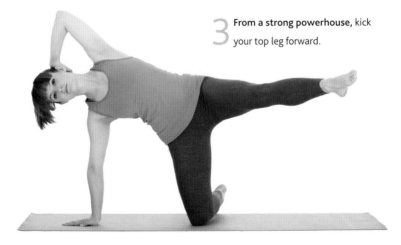

2 **Place your right hand on the mat underneath your right shoulder.** Kneel on your right knee and lift your left leg to hip height, parallel to the mat; place your left hand behind your head, with the elbow pointing to the ceiling.

3 **From a strong powerhouse,** kick your top leg forward.

4 **Now press your hips forward as you kick the leg back.** Keep the kicks small to ensure that your trunk stays still in space and a straight line is maintained between the head, shoulders and hips. Make the kicks bigger as you learn to stabilize your hips, trunk and shoulders. To progress further, add a double kick when you kick forward and back.

TRANSITION Place your left knee to the mat and your left hand on the mat underneath your shoulder, with your right hand behind your head, and your right leg at hip height. After completing this exercise on both sides, lower the top knee to the floor and sit sideways on the mat, ready for Mermaid Side Bends.

MODIFICATIONS

The Kneeling Side Kicks series is a more demanding version of the Side Kick series. **If you have weakness or an injury in your wrists, elbows or shoulders,** focus your attention instead on the Side Kick Series on pages 286–307.

COMMON ERRORS

- Top leg drifting toward the floor
- Hips and top elbow swaying around as the leg moves
- Losing the powerhouse and rib connection

INFORMATION

NUMBER OF REPETITIONS

4 kicks on each side.

CAUTIONS For fragile wrists and elbows, or recent injuries, omit this exercise and focus on the Side Kick series instead. If you are unable to kneel, do not do this exercise. For certain neck issues, ensure that you maintain your alignment, and keep your eyes fixed on a point in front of you.

VISUALIZATION Imagine that you have a rod right along your spine, from the crown of your head to the tip of your tailbone.

PRECISION POINTS

- The hips stay stacked and stable.
- The top leg stays parallel to the mat.
- The elbow stays pointing toward the ceiling, with the chest open and the neck long.
- The eyes are kept fixed on a point in front of you.
- The powerhouse stays switched on, and keeps your middle stationary.

Mermaid Side Bends

GOALS:
- ✓ Works the abdominals, particularly the oblique muscles
- ✓ Provides a dynamic stretch to the sides of the body
- ✓ Challenges balance and core strength
- ✓ Challenges dynamic stability of the shoulder blades

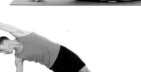

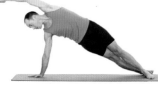

1 **Sit on the mat on your right hip, with your right hand on the mat under your right shoulder.** Slightly bend your knees, with your left foot on the mat in front of the right foot, and your left hand on your left knee, with the palm facing the ceiling.

2 **Inhale and lift your hips to the ceiling in one long line;** lift the arm in line with your ear, to feel a stretch along your side from your fingers to your toes; turn to look at your supporting hand.

3 **Exhale and lower your hips toward—but not touching—the mat;** your supporting arm should stay straight, and the underside of your body should be stretched. Lower your top arm in line with the top leg, as you turn to look at your hand as it reaches toward your toes. Inhale to lift again strongly from the hips, and reach your top arm over your ear; stretch from fingertips to toes.

TRANSITION Lower your hips to the mat, place your hands behind you on the mat and lift your legs, as one, to switch to the other side and repeat the exercise. After the last repetition, lower your hips to the mat, then face the front of the mat, with your legs extended in front of you and your ankles crossed, ready for Boomerang.

MODIFICATIONS

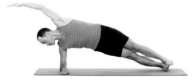

For weak wrists and elbows, weight-bear on your forearm, with your hand in front and your top foot stacked on your bottom foot.

COMMON ERRORS

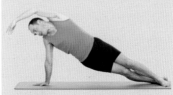

- Sinking into the wrist and shoulder
- Coming up to the lift with a ballistic movement
- The shoulders rolling forward, losing the neat, straight line of the body

INFORMATION

NUMBER OF REPETITIONS
3 lifts on each side.

....

CAUTIONS For shoulder problems, omit this exercise. For wrist and elbow problems, use the Modifications.

....

VISUALIZATION A helium balloon tied to your hips is lifting your hips up effortlessly.

PRECISION POINTS
- The top arm goes to the ear, not in front of the face.
- One long line is created, as if between two sheets of glass; there is no forward bend or rotation in the body.
- The emphasis is on the lift, but with control and precision.
- The supporting shoulder and powerhouse are kept strong throughout.

Boomerang

GOALS:
✓ Develops stamina, strength, control and coordination

✓ Cultivates flexibility in the shoulder girdle, spine and hamstrings

✓ Incorporates elements from a number of other exercises, all in one move

✓ Uses all six of the Pilates principles described on pages 24–27

1 **Sit tall on the mat with your legs out long in front and your right ankle crossed over the left, hands by hips, palms down and fingers forward.** With your abdominals in and up, lift out of your hips to sit taller.

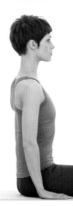

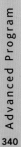

2 **Inhale, to initiate from the abdominals.** Exhale and roll back in one movement, until your legs are over your head and parallel to the floor. Do not roll onto your neck; instead press your arms firmly into the mat, so that the weight is on your shoulders and the backs of your arms.

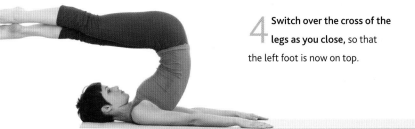

3 Inhale and open your legs hip-width apart.

4 Switch over the cross of the legs as you close, so that the left foot is now on top.

5 Exhale and roll up to the Teaser position (see page 308); with your ankles still crossed, pull in your abdominals and reach for your toes.

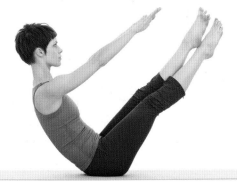

6 **Maintain your balance, inhale, turn your palms up and bend your elbows.** Reach your hands behind you and clasp them together. Reach your hands back to stretch the front of your chest, and lift tall through the crown of your head. Reach your legs away, in opposition.

7 **On the exhale, float your whole body forward and down, until your legs gently touch the mat, with your hands lifting to the ceiling;** your nose should be toward your knees, in a deep stretch.

8 **Release your hands;** circle them forward to your ankles and enjoy the deepest of stretches, then articulate your spine up to a sitting position.

TRANSITION From the sitting position, lift yourself forward on the mat to bring your buttocks to your heels, ready for Seal.

MODIFICATIONS

If you have shoulder problems or are struggling to hold the Teaser position, refrain from bringing your hands behind you; maintain the balance and lower your legs gently to the mat.

COMMON ERRORS

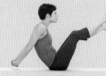

- The chin protruding when taking the arms back, and the chest and spine sinking
- Poor control when lowering the legs, causing a strain on the lower back
- Using momentum or your hands to roll back
- Rolling onto the neck
- Hearing the heels hit the mat with a thud, rather than through a controlled descent

INFORMATION

NUMBER OF REPETITIONS 4.

CAUTIONS For shoulder problems, omit taking your hands behind you and follow the modifications. For neck and lower back problems, omit this exercise.

VISUALIZATION Move through space like a boomerang; maintain the shape of the boomerang with smooth, controlled, flowing movements.

PRECISION POINTS

- The abdominals are kept engaged throughout, to keep the spine lifted.
- As you roll back the legs, go parallel with the floor; the spine stays lifted, with space between chin and chest.
- Most of the weight is on the shoulders, not the neck.
- The neck stays long throughout.
- The movement is initiated from the abdominals, with a strong centerline, for the duration of the exercise.
- Keep it moving.

Seal

GOALS:
- ✓ Improves flexibility in the hips
- ✓ Challenges balance and coordination
- ✓ Works the abdominals to control movement and prevent the use of momentum
- ✓ Acts as a cool-down at the end of the mat-work

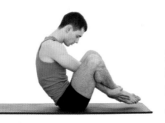

1 **Sitting toward the front edge of your mat, simultaneously move your hands between your legs and tip back to balance on your sit-bones, with your abdominals pulled in.** Your knees should be shoulder-width apart as your elbows press out to your knees. You have come into a balance in a tight shape, held steady and controlled by an active scoop. Your arms and legs should be active, with your shoulders away from your ears. Clap your feet together 3 times.

2 **Inhale and, working from your abdominals, roll back to the base of your shoulder blades.** Balance on the back of your shoulders and clap your feet together 3 times.

3 **Exhale and, with control, roll up to the starting position.** Balance, then clap your feet together 3 times.

TRANSITION On the last roll let go of your ankles in the backward position, place one ankle over the other, feet to the floor, and spring into a standing position as you roll forward, ready for Push-Ups.

COMMON ERRORS

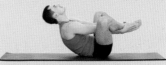

- Initiating the movement from the head by tipping it back
- Losing the Seal shape of the exercise, so that the feet come away from the seat, the knees fall out of the frame and the chin comes away from the chest
- Poor control from the powerhouse, so that the head lands on the mat in the backward position and the feet hit the floor in front

MODIFICATIONS

If you have a stiff lower back, or your wrists and elbows are uncomfortable in the full position, place your hands on the back of your thighs.

INFORMATION

NUMBER OF REPETITIONS 6–8.

CAUTIONS Those with osteoporosis and disc problems should omit this exercise. With hip replacements, proceed with caution until the hips are really strong. Use the Modifications if the full position strains the wrists and elbows.

VISUALIZATION Roll like a seal.

PRECISION POINTS
- The elbows press out, the knees press in.
- Keep the Seal shape: chin to chest, heels toward the seat, and eyes locked on your middle.
- Exhale as you roll up with a strong controlled scoop.
- As you clap your feet in the backward roll, hold the balance for a moment.

Push-Ups

GOALS:
✓ Strengthens and stabilizes the shoulders and upper back
✓ Tones and strengthens the arms, with specific focus on the triceps
✓ Trains strength and stability of the core

1 **Stand in the Pilates stance at the end of your mat;** inhale to lift your hands to the ceiling.

2 **Exhale and lift your abdominals to start to roll down, as if peeling away from a wall, until your hands reach the mat with your legs straight;** keep your weight forward, so that you don't press your weight back behind your heels.

3 For a count of 1, step your left hand out halfway along the mat; for a count of 2, step your right hand past the left to your full length; and for a count of 3, bring your left hand level with the right hand, to make a Front Support position (see page 204).

4 Inhale to dip at the elbows, keeping them so close to the body that your elbows shave your ribs. Exhale and press up in one strong line; repeat 3 times.

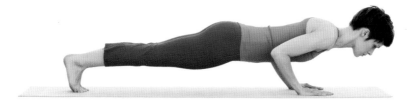

5 **After the last push-up, lift your hips to the ceiling;** push down through your hands and heels, to feel a deep stretch. Step one hand back half the distance toward your feet; step the other hand back to your feet, then the first hand joins it. Roll up to a standing position, using your powerhouse to articulate your spine upward, as if rolling up against a wall, and taking your arms overhead. Roll down for another set of Push-Ups.

TRANSITION You have finished the Pilates mat workout! Stand tall and proud in the Pilates stance.

MODIFICATIONS

If you are unable to hold the Front Support position, or do a push-up without sinking in the shoulders or lower back/hips, bend your knees to the mat, bring your heels to your backside and weight-bear through the front of your thighs (not the kneecaps).

For weak arms, keep the movement in the push-up small, until you are strong enough to dip further.

COMMON ERRORS

- Sinking into the shoulders, with the chin poking out
- The lower back and hips sinking as you dip in the push-up
- The hips lifted toward the ceiling
- The head hanging between the shoulders

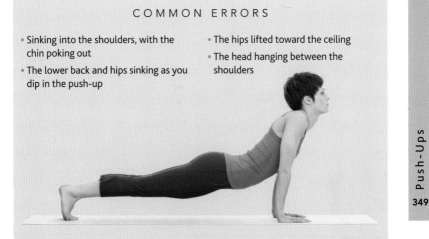

INFORMATION

NUMBER OF REPETITIONS

3 sets of 3 push-ups.

CAUTIONS For wrist, elbow or shoulder problems, proceed with caution. For weak abdominals, shoulders or back problems, use the first Modification.

VISUALIZATION Adopt a solid plank position and maintain it throughout the exercise.

PRECISION POINTS

- The arms press into the sides, with the elbows pointing to the heels.
- The shoulders are engaged down the back; think about turning your shoulder blades in slightly; line up the middle finger with the center of your wrist, to help engage the shoulders in the right place.
- Hands are under shoulders, toes under heels.
- The centerline connection is worked by zipping the legs together.

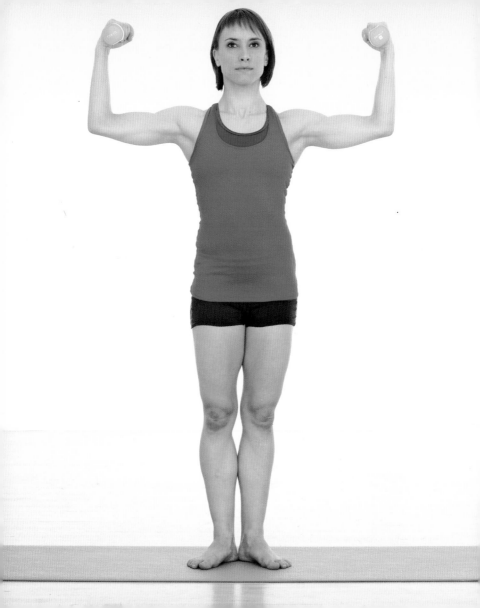

Arm-Weight Series

The Arm-Weight Series brings you into a standing position to work your powerhouse. Your core is challenged to keep you stable while you are up against gravity; you need to apply the same principles as when working on the mat.

"Standing also is very important and should be practiced at all times until it is mastered . . . never slouch, as doing so compresses the lungs, overcrowds other vital organs, rounds the back and throws off the balance." JOSEPH PILATES

Standing Arm-Weight Series

The body's deep core muscles are designed to maintain our posture against gravity when we are upright, as this is where we spend most of our waking day: sitting, standing, walking, moving around. The Standing Arm-Weight Series is an opportunity to train the deep core muscles to stabilize the trunk, supported by the muscles of the hips, the pelvis and the shoulder girdle.

In these exercises, focus on finding a good posture— with your weight evenly distributed over the four corners of your feet, knees over ankles, hips over knees, shoulders over hips and your eyes to the horizon, the back of your neck lengthened and your powerhouse pulled in and up.

You can use hand-weights to provide light resistance: 1 lb (0.5 kg), 2 lb (1 kg) or 3 lb (1.5 kg) weights. Equally you can practice the Standing Arm-Weight Series without weights, using self-resistance, focusing on your posture and the quality of your movements. There are two starting positions, as follows.

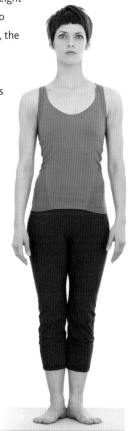

PILATES STANCE

Ensure that you are aligned in a standing position, as described above. When you stand with the back of your thighs and your seat wrapped, your feet will naturally take on a slight turn-out.

TABLETOP POSITION

Stand with your feet parallel and underneath your hips, knees over toes. Bend at the hips and pull your powerhouse in, to bring your spine to a flat tabletop position. Your head should be in line with your spine.

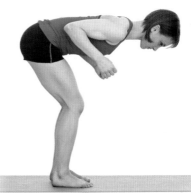

GOALS:
- ✓ Promotes stability of the trunk
- ✓ Teaches core control in standing
- ✓ Strengthens and tones all the major muscle groups of the arms, shoulders and upper back
- ✓ Trains the muscles that stabilize the shoulder blades on the back, while the arms move
- ✓ Different arm-weight exercises variously mobilize the shoulders, the front of the chest and the upper spine

CAUTIONS

The Standing Arm-Weight Series is appropriate at every level, from beginner's to advanced, and is suitable for almost everybody. However, there are a few considerations over which to exercise caution, as follows:

- **For neck or shoulder pain,** work within your pain-free range and without weights. You may even have to omit this series.

- **For wrist and elbow problems,** proceed with caution; try working without weights initially.

Biceps I

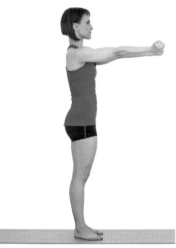 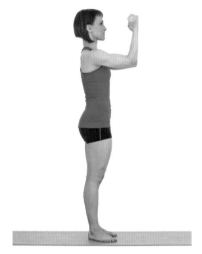

1 **Stand in the Pilates stance, with your arms out in front at shoulder height**. Hold the weights, with your palms facing the ceiling.

2 **Slowly bend your elbows to bring your hands to your shoulders.** Slowly straighten your elbows back to the starting position.

DO 3–5 repetitions.
* Focus on your posture.
* Scoop, and grow taller with each repetition.
* Resist as you bend the elbows, resist as you straighten the elbows.

* Keep the shoulder blades sliding down your back.
* Breathe naturally.
....
DON'T Let the elbows drop as you bend and straighten—they should stay level with the shoulders.

Biceps II

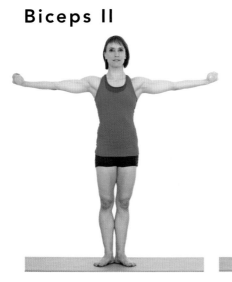

1 **Stand in the Pilates stance, with your arms out to the side at shoulder height and your hands in the periphery of your vision.** Hold the weights, with your palms facing the ceiling.

2 **Slowly bend your elbows to bring your hands to your shoulders.** Slowly straighten your elbows back to the starting position.

DO 3–5 repetitions.
* Focus on your posture.
* Scoop, and grow taller with each repetition.
* Resist as you bend the elbows, resist as you straighten the elbows.

* Keep the shoulder blades sliding down the back.
* Breathe naturally.

DON'T Let the elbows drop as you bend and straighten—they should stay level with the shoulders.

Biceps III

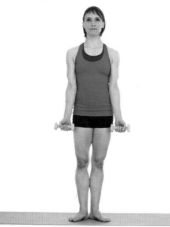

1 **Stand in the Pilates stance,** with your arms by your side and your palms facing forward.

2 **Slowly bend your elbows to a 90° angle.** Then slowly straighten them to return to your starting position.

DO 3–5 repetitions.
- Scoop, and grow taller with each repetition.
- Resist as you bend the elbows, resist as you straighten the elbows.
- Keep the shoulder blades sliding down the back.
- Keep the collarbone soft and open, with the elbows and wrists in line with the shoulders.

- Focus on your posture.
- Breathe naturally.

DON'T
- Throw the hips forward when bending the arms.
- Let the shoulders roll forward.
- Lose the scoop and stand with a protruding belly and a poking chin.

Triceps

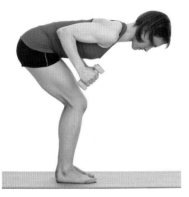

1 **Start in the tabletop position.** Bend your elbows and press them tightly into your side. Hold the weights so that your palms are facing one another.

2 **Press your hands back toward the ceiling,** so that your elbows straighten without moving from their position. Bend the elbows to bring your hands back to the starting position.

DO 3–5 repetitions.
- Scoop deeper, and lengthen the spine longer with each repetition.
- Resist to straighten, resist to bend.
- Keep the elbows steady and pressed into your sides.

- Breathe naturally.

DON'T Let the elbows move around.

Side Stretch

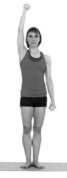

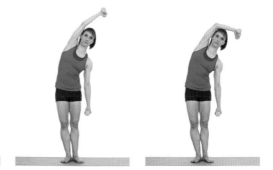

1 **Start in the Pilates stance,** with your arms by your sides and your palms facing in. Bend your right elbow and take the arm toward the ceiling alongside your right ear.

2 **Inhale, scoop and bend to your left.** Bend the elbow to reach toward the opposite ear. Straighten the elbow, reaching to the opposite wall. Return to the center, and bring your arm back to your side. Switch arms and repeat.

DO 3–5 repetitions each side.
- Keep the powerhouse engaged throughout.
- Keep both heels firmly planted into the floor.
- Keep the pelvis square and the eyes facing forward.
- Lengthen your side as you reach over to the opposite wall.
- Keep both sides long as you bend to the side.

DON'T
- Let the hips slide out to the side as you reach away.
- Let the heel lift off the floor as you reach away.

Boxing

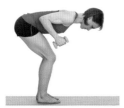 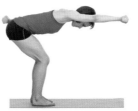 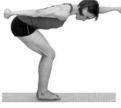

1 **Start in the tabletop position.** Bend your elbows and press them tightly into your sides. Hold the weights with your palms facing one another.

2 **Inhale and straighten one arm in front,** in line with your ear, palm down—the other arm should lengthen behind, palm up. Exhale and return to the starting position.

3 **Inhale and repeat by switching arms.**

DO 3–5 repetitions.
- Lengthen the arms away in opposition, with a strong powerhouse.
- Keep the spine lengthened.
- Keep the arms in line with the head and the body as you reach away.
- Move slowly, and in a controlled way.

DON'T
- Let the arms flail around!
- Let the back sink or arch.

Chest Expansion

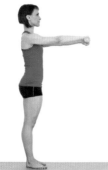

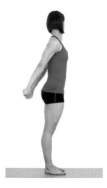

1 **Stand in the Pilates stance.** Your arms should be at shoulder height in front, with the weights in your hands and your palms facing down. Your powerhouse should be pulled in and up, with the back of your neck lengthened so that the crown of your head reaches toward the ceiling.

2 **Inhale and press your hands back behind you, arms skimming your sides.** Turn your head to the right, through the center and then to the left.

3 **Exhale as you turn your head back to the center** and return your arms to shoulder height.

DO 2–4 repetitions on each side.
• Slide the shoulder blades down your back as you press the arms behind you.
• Let the front of the chest open, and the neck grow long.

• Let the in-breath grow as you press the arms back and turn the head.
• Keep the ribs flush with your front.

DON'T
• Let the chin poke forward.

Zip Up

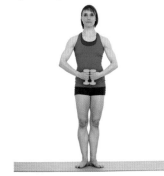

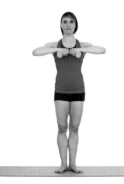

1 **Stand in the Pilates stance**, with your hands in front of your hips and palms facing you.

2 **Inhale and lift your weights up the center of your body, bending your elbows out to the side.** Exhale and resist, as you press the weights back to the starting position. As an added challenge, lift up onto your toes, keeping your heels together as you press the weights down; lower back onto your heels as you raise the weights.

DO 5 repetitions.
* "Zip up" all your connections as you lift the weights: inner thigh, scoop, ribs flattening and shoulder blades sliding down the back.

DON'T
* Let the shoulders lift to your ears as you lift the weights.

Sparklers (Arm Circles)

1–2 **Stand in the Pilates stance,** holding the weights by their ends in front of your hips. Bring the weights in front of you.

3–4 **Breathing naturally,** make steady circular movements, keeping your arms straight, and begin to move your arms up in front of you.

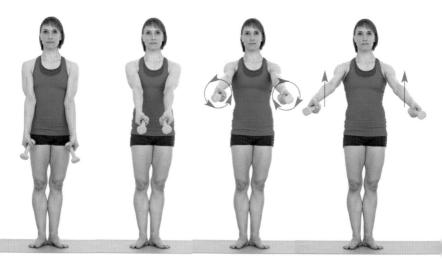

DO 3–5 repetitions up and down.

• Keep the powerhouse lifted throughout, to keep you lifted and tall.

• Keep the shoulder blades down.

• Keep the arms aligned from the shoulders, through the elbows to the wrists.

• Circle the arms from the shoulders, without moving the wrists and hands.

• Keep your weight forward over your toes, and use your powerhouse to keep you balanced.

DON'T

• Let your middle and hips move around as you circle the arms.

• Let the shoulders lift to the ears as the arms circle upward.

5–6 Do eight circles to take the arms up.

7–8 At the top, do eight reverse circles to lower your arms back down.

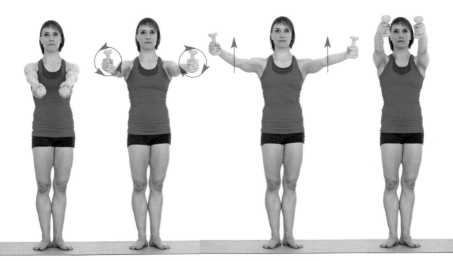

Ten-Minute and Entire Mat Workouts

Joseph Pilates was adamant that practice was vital to gain the maximum benefit from his system. He advocated that doing ten minutes well on his routine was more effective than doing a longer time badly, or not doing it at all.

This chapter gives one short workout and the entire mat sequence that enable you to achieve the benefits of Pilates. However, don't be tempted to practice just the exercises that you like or the ones that feel easy! When you follow the set Pilates order, most areas of your fitness will be challenged: flexibility, strength, stability, stamina and coordination. If you cherry-pick a few exercises, then you are likely to miss some of these important components. Pilates also intended his system to challenge the cardiovascular system, and if you work with flow in the ten-minute workout and in the entire sequence you will raise your heart rate.

"Make up your mind that you will perform your Pilates exercise ten minutes without fail." JOSEPH PILATES

Two-Rep Drill

This drill consists of 27 exercises and will only take ten minutes. Do not be tempted to sacrifice precision and control for speed; keep focused and you can remain true to the Pilates principles.

Follow the Intermediate Program (see pages 128–211) and add the Push-Up series from the Advanced Program; however, rather than completing the full set of repetitions, stick to just two repetitions of each exercise. Execute clean, neat Transitions and go on to the next move, creating a sense of flow. Afterward you should feel energized, stretched and ready to face the world. Here is the list of exercises that comprise the Two-Rep Drill:

EXERCISE

1 The Hundred (pages 130–1)

2 Roll Up (pages 132–5)

3 One-Leg Circles (pages 136–9)

4 Rolling Like a Ball (pages 140–1)

Abdominal Five series:

5 • Single Leg Stretch (pages 142–3)

6 • Double Leg Stretch (pages 144–5)

7 • Single Straight-Leg Stretch 'Scissors' (pages 146–7)

8 • Double Straight-Leg Stretch 'Lower Lifts' (pages 148–51)

9 • Criss-Cross (pages 152–3)

10 Spine Stretch Forward (pages 154–7)

11 Open-Leg Rocker—Preparation (pages 158–61)

12 Corkscrew I (pages 162–5)

13 Saw (pages 166–7)

14 Swan Neck Roll (pages 168–9) + Rest Position (page 170)

15 Shoulder Bridge Preparation (pages 172–5)

Side Kick series:

16 • Front/Back (pages 176–9)

17 • Up/Down (pages 180–1)

18 • Passé (pages 182–5)

19 • Circles (pages 186–7)

20 • Inner Thigh Lifts and Circles (pages 188–91)

21 Teaser 1 Leg (pages 192–5)

22 Teaser 1 (pages 196–9)

23 Swimming (pages 200–3)

24 Leg Pull Front Support (pages 204–5)

25 Mermaid (pages 206–9)

26 Seal (pages 210–11)

27 Push-Up series (pages 346–9)

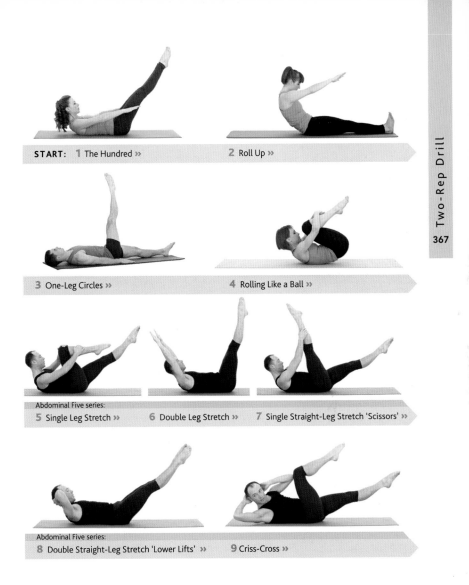

START: 1 The Hundred »

2 Roll Up »

3 One-Leg Circles »

4 Rolling Like a Ball »

Abdominal Five series:
5 Single Leg Stretch » 6 Double Leg Stretch » 7 Single Straight-Leg Stretch 'Scissors' »

Abdominal Five series:
8 Double Straight-Leg Stretch 'Lower Lifts' » 9 Criss-Cross »

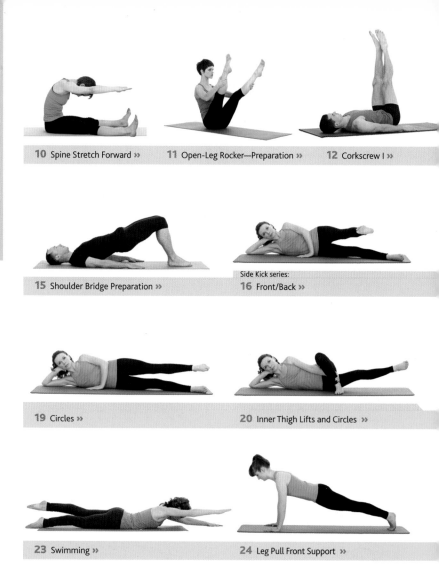

10 Spine Stretch Forward »   **11** Open-Leg Rocker—Preparation »   **12** Corkscrew I »

15 Shoulder Bridge Preparation »

Side Kick series:
16 Front/Back »

19 Circles »

20 Inner Thigh Lifts and Circles »

23 Swimming »

24 Leg Pull Front Support »

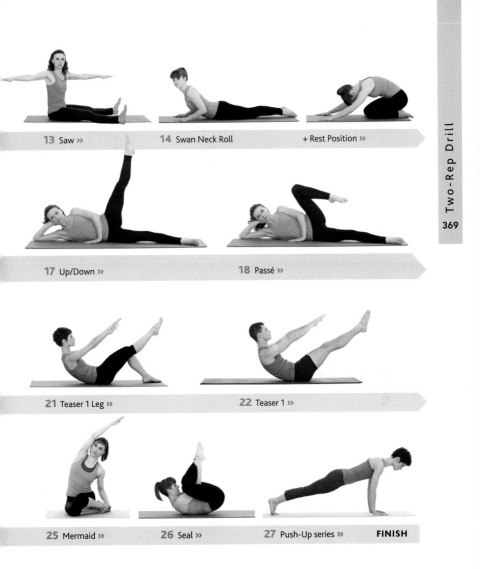

13 Saw »   **14** Swan Neck Roll   + Rest Position »

17 Up/Down »   **18** Passé »

21 Teaser 1 Leg »   **22** Teaser 1 »

25 Mermaid »   **26** Seal »   **27** Push-Up series »   **FINISH**

Entire Mat Sequence

"If you faithfully perform your Pilates exercises regularly only four times a week for just three months . . . you will find your body development approaching the ideal, accompanied by renewed mental vigour and spiritual enhancement." JOSEPH PILATES

This section provides you with a tool to assist you in practicing Pilates. Here you will find, in sequential order, the entire mat workout from the Intermediate and Advanced programs, illustrated with pictures to prompt your memory, accompanied by the maximum number of repetitions, to prompt you and keep you moving as you practice.

Follow the order of the exercises, work with precision and use the Transitions between exercises that you learned from the more detailed descriptions earlier on, to ensure that you flow smoothly from one exercise to the next. Exclude any exercises that are not appropriate for your body, and remember to use any Modifications that you require. Now get practicing!

	EXERCISE	MAXIMUM NUMBER OF REPETITIONS
1	The Hundred (pages 214–17)	100 pumps, 10 breaths
2	Roll Up (pages 218–21)	5
3	Roll Over (pages 222–5)	3 in each direction
4	One-Leg Circles (pages 226–9)	5 each way on each leg
5	Rolling like a Ball (pages 230–1)	8 repetitions
	Abdominal Five series:	
6	• Single Leg Stretch (pages 232–3)	10
7	• Double Leg Stretch (pages 234–5)	10
8	• Single Straight-Leg Stretch 'Scissors' (pages 236–7)	10
9	• Double Straight-Leg Stretch 'Lower Lifts' (pages 238–41)	10
10	• Criss-Cross (pages 242–3)	10
11	Spine Stretch Forward (pages 244–7)	5

	EXERCISE	MAXIMUM NUMBER OF REPETITIONS
12	Open-Leg Rocker (pages 248–51)	8
13	Corkscrew I (pages 162–5)	4 in each direction
14	Corkscrew II (pages 252–53)	4 in each direction
15	Saw (pages 254–7)	5
16	Swan Neck Roll (pages 168–71)	2 with the neck roll, 1 lift to the center
17	Swan Dive (pages 258–61)	5
18	Single Leg Kicks (pages 262–3)	5 on each leg
19	Double Leg Kicks (pages 264–5)	3 sets
20	Rest Position (page 170)	–
21	Neck Pull (pages 266–9)	5
22	Scissors (Shoulder Stand) (pages 270–1)	3 on each leg
23	Bicycles (Shoulder Stand) (pages 272–5)	3 sets in each direction
24	Shoulder Bridge Preparation (pages 172–5)	5 lifts of the pelvis; 3 lifts on each leg if doing the progression
25	Shoulder Bridge (pages 276–9)	3 lifts on each leg
26	Spine Twist (pages 280–1)	3 each way
27	Jackknife (pages 282–5)	3
	Side Kick series:	
28	• Front/Back (pages 286–9)	10
29	• Up/Down (pages 290–1)	5
30	• Passé (pages 292–3)	3 each way on each leg
31	• Circles (pages 294–5)	8
32	• Inner Thigh Lifts and Circles (pages 296–7)	8
33	• Hot Potato (pages 298–9)	4 sets of heel taps and kicks
34	• Grande Ronde de Jambe (pages 300–3)	3 each way
35	• Bicycle (pages 304–7)	3 each way
36	Beats on the Belly Transition (page 190)	10 counts
37	Teaser 1 (pages 308–11)	3
38	Teaser II (pages 312–13)	3
39	Teaser III (pages 314–15)	3
40	Cancan (pages 316–19)	3
41	Hip Circles (pages 320–3)	3 sets of circles in each direction
42	Swimming (pages 324–5)	2 sets of inhale/exhale
43	Leg Pull Front (pages 326–9)	3 on each leg
44	Leg Pull Up (pages 330–3)	3 on each leg
45	Kneeling Side Kick series (pages 334–7)	4 kicks on each side
46	Mermaid Side Bends (pages 338–9)	3 lifts on each side
47	Boomerang (pages 340–3)	4
48	Seal (pages 344–5)	8
49	Push-Ups (pages 346–9)	3 sets of 3 push-ups

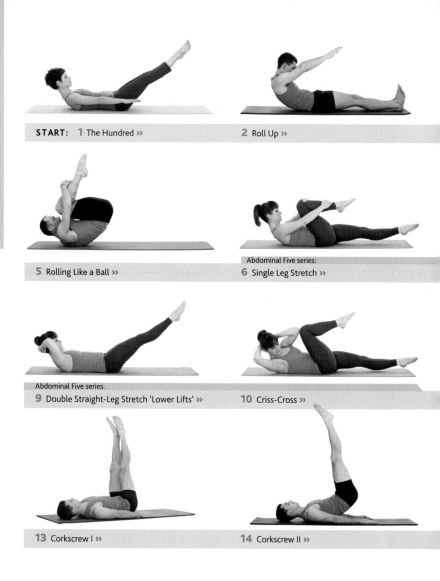

START: **1** The Hundred »

2 Roll Up »

5 Rolling Like a Ball »

Abdominal Five series:
6 Single Leg Stretch »

Abdominal Five series:
9 Double Straight-Leg Stretch 'Lower Lifts' »

10 Criss-Cross »

13 Corkscrew I »

14 Corkscrew II »

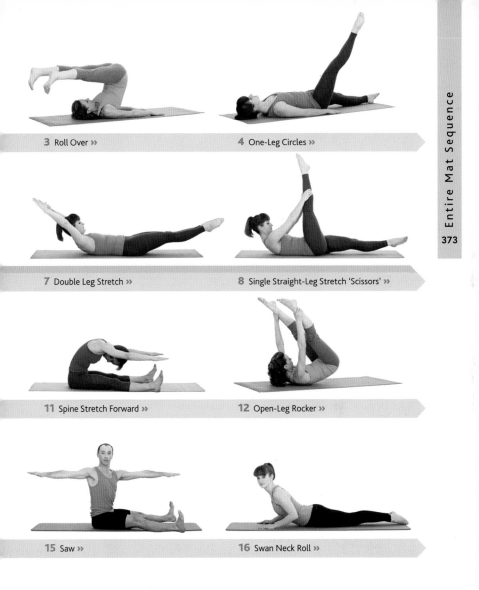

3 Roll Over »

4 One-Leg Circles »

7 Double Leg Stretch »

8 Single Straight-Leg Stretch 'Scissors' »

11 Spine Stretch Forward »

12 Open-Leg Rocker »

15 Saw »

16 Swan Neck Roll »

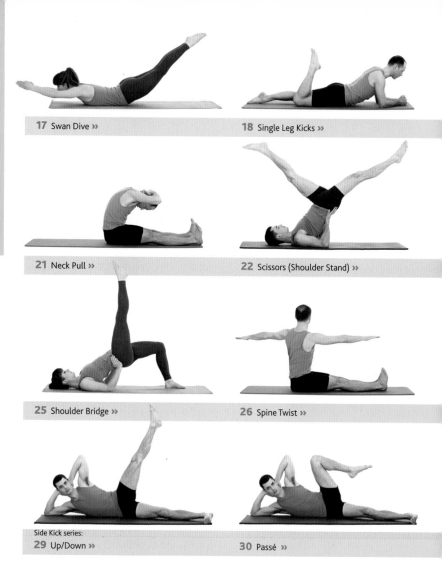

17 Swan Dive »

18 Single Leg Kicks »

21 Neck Pull »

22 Scissors (Shoulder Stand) »

25 Shoulder Bridge »

26 Spine Twist »

Side Kick series:
29 Up/Down »

30 Passé »

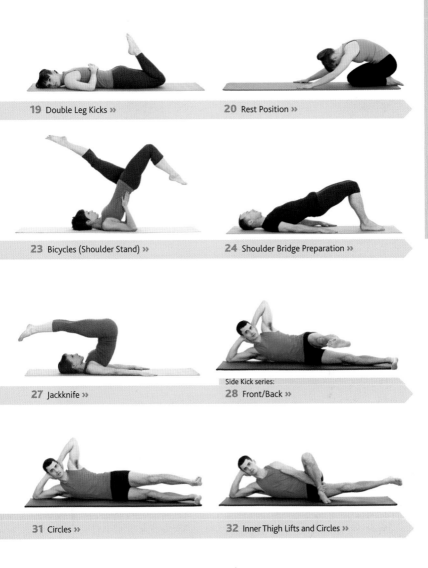

19 Double Leg Kicks »

20 Rest Position »

23 Bicycles (Shoulder Stand) »

24 Shoulder Bridge Preparation »

27 Jackknife »

Side Kick series:
28 Front/Back »

31 Circles »

32 Inner Thigh Lifts and Circles »

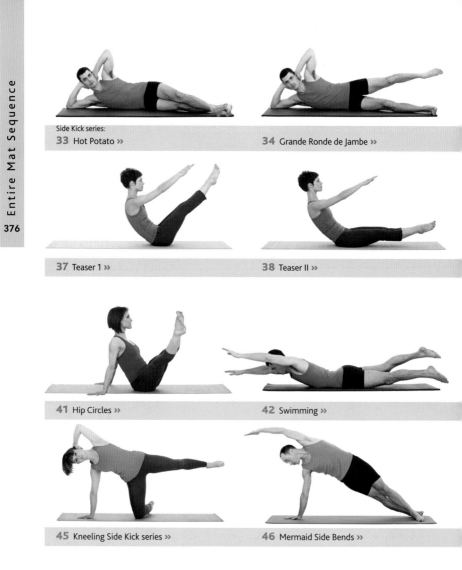

Side Kick series:
33 Hot Potato »

34 Grande Ronde de Jambe »

37 Teaser 1 »

38 Teaser II »

41 Hip Circles »

42 Swimming »

45 Kneeling Side Kick series »

46 Mermaid Side Bends »

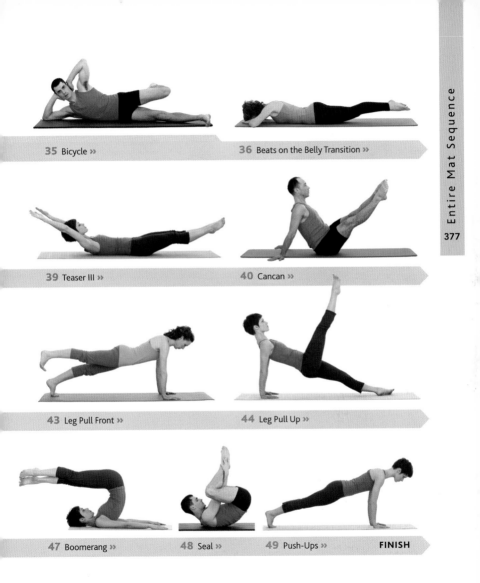

35 Bicycle »

36 Beats on the Belly Transition »

39 Teaser III »

40 Cancan »

43 Leg Pull Front »

44 Leg Pull Up »

47 Boomerang »

48 Seal »

49 Push-Ups »

FINISH

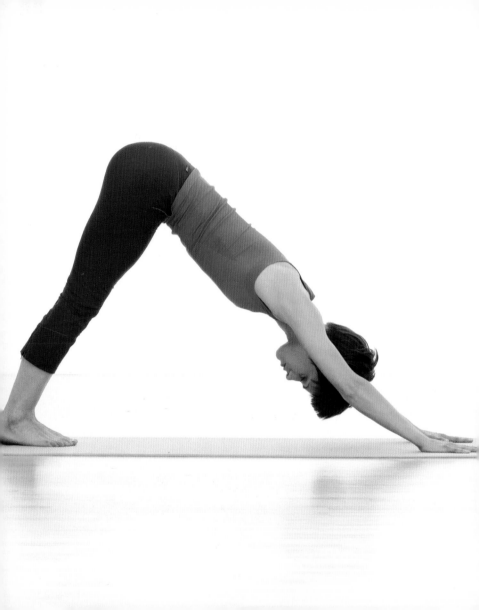

Pilates in Your Everyday Life

As your fitness and your body awareness increase with practice, you will feel the changes in your body while you are carrying out the exercises. The next step is to use these principles as part of your daily routine.

"Pilates develops the body uniformly, corrects wrong postures, restores vitality, invigorates the mind, and elevates the spirit."
JOSEPH PILATES

Posture and Movement

"Good posture can be successfully acquired only when the entire mechanism of the body is under perfect control. Graceful carriage follows as a matter of course." JOSEPH PILATES

Good posture has far more significance than simply pleasing those in your life who might have nagged you as a child to "Sit up tall/stand straight!" Good posture is a sign of a healthy body, with minimal restrictions and limitations in the joints, muscles and ligaments, and with good core control.

A healthy postural alignment means being able to achieve, and sustain, the following:

- The three normal curves in the spine: namely, the natural hollows in the neck and lower back and a gentle rounding in the thoracic spine
- Alignment in the horizontal plane: both ears, shoulders, hips, knees and ankles level with each other
- Alignment in the centerline: nose over breastbone, and both of these aligned in turn over the pubic bone
- Alignment in the anterior/posterior plane: knees over ankles, hips over knees, shoulders directly over pelvis, and head sitting balanced on top of the neck, with the eyes level with the horizon
- Even distribution of weight over both feet, with the plumb line falling just in front of the ankles and equidistant between both feet.

The muscles of the powerhouse act very much like a traditional corset, supporting the spine between the pelvis and ribs. When the powerhouse is active, it should aid in unloading or decompressing the spine when the body is static, walking around, twisting and bending. If the spine is not adequately supported by the deep core muscles, then the discs and joints in the spine can experience far more compression and load. This is further compounded by twisting, bending, extending the spine or adopting prolonged poor postures.

POOR POSTURE

Adopting poor postures repetitively over time will cause restrictions, limitations and eventually pain within your body.

Carrying the Pilates principles from the mat-work into your everyday life can have an instant beneficial impact on your posture and body. You can find your scoop (and engage your powerhouse and other connections) while standing waiting for the kettle to boil, sitting at your desk, walking around the office at work or bending to pick up something from the floor. This action will lift and lengthen your spine and lighten the way you feel; it may even raise your energy levels. Using your powerhouse when engaging in exercise such as running, walking or cycling will protect your spine, help to engage your pelvic floor and give you a boost that will supply an additional burst of energy.

GOOD POSTURE

Good posture will help maintain healthy joints and a healthy spine as well as make you appear energized and youthful.

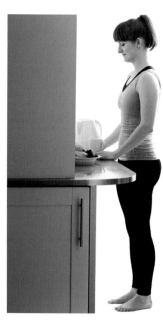
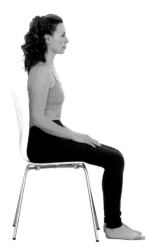

SWITCHING ON YOUR POWERHOUSE
IN EVERYDAY LIFE

Before you start practicing Pilates, the area of the body known as the powerhouse is not something you are likely to be aware of. By actively beginning to use your powerhouse throughout the day, you increase your awareness of that part of your body. This in turn leads to an increase in mindfulness; you become better tuned into your body, how it feels and where it is in space—more aware of less desirable postures, and in turn able to move better and adopt better postures. Being more mindful of your body develops the habit of the powerhouse becoming active spontaneously, rather than through conscious thought, and creates a body that is less prone to pain and injury—not forgetting the enhanced sense of well-being that it provides.

Pilates, therefore, is not just something to follow when you are on your exercise mat; use your powerhouse and the Pilates principles as you go about your everyday life and you will reap many benefits. Naturally these benefits will be all the more valuable if your lifestyle includes enough sleep, sufficient exercise and a healthy diet.

Pilates for Special Circumstances

This book contains many adaptations of exercises for different health issues, but space does not permit offering specialized Pilates workouts for every type of health condition or consideration, which would also require individual assessment of the person in question. So here are some general guidelines to using Pilates when recovering from injury or if you have current health problems:

- *Always* consult your healthcare professional—your doctor, physical therapist, chiropractor or osteopath, or whoever is involved in managing your health—before embarking on Pilates or returning to it after an injury.
- Seek out a Pilates instructor who has trained through a recognized institution, and who has experience in teaching Pilates to individuals with health difficulties.
- Consider visiting an instructor for individual sessions, as opposed to attending a class. This does have cost implications, but the benefits will be worth the financial outlay. You will be able to work toward specific goals that are set by your instructor and focus your Pilates workout on your individual needs.
- Develop body awareness, so that you are mindful of what is happening in your body—*never* work through pain.
- Learn the Fundamentals in Chapter 3 (see pages 58–83).
- Then start your practice with the Beginner's Program (see pages 84–127).
- Use the Modifications that are appropriate for you, which have been given in the instructions for each exercise.
- Always work within your own capabilities.

Now let's look at recommendations for particular health conditions.

LOWER BACK PAIN

There are many reasons why people suffer from back pain, such as postural causes, injury, wear and tear or disease. Frequently the pain is due to poor posture and subsequent changes in the structure and alignment of the muscles, ligaments and bones. Back pain that is due to postural problems responds well to Pilates.

Remember that your abdominal muscles support your spine. When doing an exercise lying on your back, the further you lower your legs or reach them away from your body, the more you load your spine—and the greater the demand on your abdominal muscles. If you have a back problem, your abdominal muscles will perhaps already be weaker; so don't lower your legs very far, and keep your movements controlled and close to your body, to minimize the load on your spine. Keep your abdominals engaged during your workout, and support your powerhouse with the other connections in your body—the wrap of your backside and thighs, and your rib and shoulder blade connection. The safest position to start exercising in is lying on your back, with your knees bent; when you are ready to include bigger, more challenging moves, then a good instructor can guide you. Bending and rotating movements will need to be incorporated with care and guidance, when your body is ready.

NECK PROBLEMS

Pain from neck problems is common and can lead to other unpleasant symptoms, including headaches and muscle tension. When doing Pilates exercises lying on a mat, the head is frequently held up, but if this causes you pain, keep your head down—in this position the back of the neck should remain lengthened; imagine reaching the crown of your head toward the wall behind you. If the back of your neck is tight, that will prevent you being able to do this; your chin will tip toward the ceiling, and the back of your neck will remain scrunched up. Use a block or a small pillow under your head; experiment with the height of the block or pillow until the back of your neck feels longer and your chin tilts slightly toward your chest.

When lying flat, a tight neck will cause your chin to poke to the ceiling and will compress the joints in your neck, which is an undesirable position.

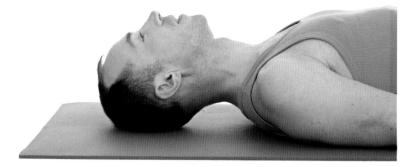

If your abdominal muscles are not strong enough for a particular exercise, the tendency will be to brace your body using your head and neck. This can also cause considerable strain and may lead to neck pain.

During the mat workout you will lie on your front and side, as well as on your back. If you have neck pain, you need to support your head so that your neck is lengthened and in line with the rest of your spine, and should avoid bracing and straining your neck.

To find the optimum position for your head and neck it may be necessary to use a block to lengthen the back of the neck.

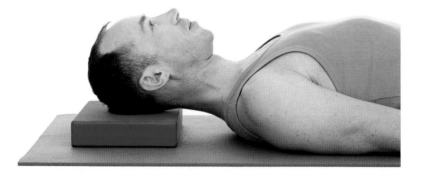

Pilates at Different Stages of Life

Just as you can vary your approach to Pilates depending on your health situation, so you can vary it at different stages of your life, such as during pregnancy and when you are younger or older.

PREGNANCY

Pilates has become popular in pregnancy, not only as a safe method of exercising, but as a form of exercise that will particularly benefit a woman's body while it changes during the months of pregnancy. However, there are some very important considerations when exercising, due to the associated changes that occur in the body:

- A hormone called relaxin is released from the time of conception and stays in a woman's body for a period of time after childbirth. Relaxin helps to soften the ligaments and other connective tissue to enable the pelvic bones to move in relation to one another and to allow the passage of the baby through the pelvic opening during childbirth. However, relaxin does not just affect the ligaments of the pelvic bones, but all the ligaments of the body, thereby increasing the risk of injury and instability. Overzealous or poorly instructed stretching or high-impact exercise, or poor posture or alignment while exercising can considerably increase the risk of injury to the pregnant woman. Exercising during pregnancy needs to be mindful of the effects that relaxin has on the body, so as to prevent injury.
- Later on during pregnancy lying flat on your back can cause dizziness, due to the baby's weight compressing some major blood vessels, which can impede the return of blood to the heart. This can happen as the baby begins to grow and the bump starts to expand and is no longer low in the pelvis, and can occur from the beginning of the second trimester. Exercising lying on your back is generally considered safe in the first trimester, but is not recommended after that.

- The change in shape in a woman's body has an impact on her posture and on the alignment of her spine and pelvis. The growing bump and larger breasts can cause a greater hollow in the lower back (known as lordosis), rounded shoulders and a pelvis that tilts forward. With the added weight, these postural changes can lead to strain on the joints, muscles and ligaments; and, with the additional effect of the hormone relaxin, some women struggle with back, pelvic and joint pain. The change in a woman's body also limits the positions that she can exercise in.

Pilates mat-work in its pure form is not really something for a pregnant woman to take up as a new form of exercise. If you are an already established student of Pilates, then it may be possible to continue with a qualified instructor for the first trimester, and then with modifications after that period. But if you wish to go to a class as a new student it is imperative to attend a specialized class and to find an instructor who has the training and knowledge to exercise women safely during pregnancy. Nevertheless there are components of the Pilates system that are positively beneficial to the pregnant body, and specialist Pilates-based post-natal classes may be enjoyable and beneficial.

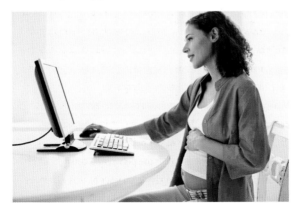

Pilates during pregnancy under the tutorship of a specialized instructor can offer a pregnant woman many benefits.

THE YOUNGER PERSON/TEENAGER

Joseph Pilates felt quite passionately that society was doing children and young people a disservice by imposing the constraints of modern life upon them, leading to sedentary lifestyles and poor posture from a young age. It was his ambition that his exercise system would be taught to children, to prevent them adopting the ills of modern life early on and carrying them through into adulthood.

There is now a great deal of emphasis on children exercising and being active, due to the rise in obesity levels in children. Pilates has so much to offer the developing body, and trains all aspects of fitness in a controlled way, in line with what we know about how children should exercise. Young people and teenagers can gain the following benefits from Pilates:

- **FLEXIBILITY:** Pilates trains flexibility in a controlled manner. As children naturally have very mobile joints, they don't need to be encouraged to adopt extreme ranges of movement. However, through various stages of their development an element of flexibility work is important, as different structures grow at different rates.

- **MUSCLE BALANCE:** Pilates aims to encourage symmetrical alignment and to counteract any muscle imbalances before they become fixed. Postural problems can be seen as early as the teenage years, due to prolonged poor posture during intensive periods of study, sports that encourage a one-sided dominance (such as hockey and tennis) and sustained periods of time on computer/video games.

- **STAMINA:** Pilates helps to promote stamina, which is unfortunately an area of fitness that suffers from the impact of a sedentary way of life.

- **CONCENTRATION, AND THE CONNECTION OF THE MIND AND BODY:** Teaching body awareness develops an enhanced sense of self, and fosters self-esteem and a positive self-image.

The teenage years are a good stage at which to start Pilates, and to be able to grasp the connection between practicing Pilates and seeing and feeling the benefits.

THE OLDER ADULT

Pilates is a low-impact form of exercise, so it has a lot to offer the older body, as there is minimum strain on the joints, as can occur in the weight-bearing and repetitive impact seen in other exercise programs. With its emphasis on controlled movement, Pilates trains strength in the muscles to help support the joints, rather than load the joints and cause further strain.

We know that, as we get older, muscle mass and strength are lost in strategic muscle groups—especially when combined with inactivity. Loss of muscle strength leads to a characteristic muscle imbalance, associated with a stooped posture, rounded shoulders and upper spine, a poking chin and tight neck, and a flat lower back—all resulting in some loss of height. However, there is also strong and positive evidence that strength-training is effective in the older adult, and indeed that some loss of muscle mass and strength is reversible—a very compelling reason to keep active and keep moving!

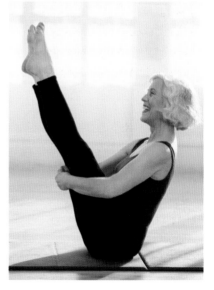

Pilates, by its very nature, helps to retrain muscle imbalances, works to counteract a stooping posture and create length and height throughout the body. So it is a highly beneficial form of exercise for the older person, when applied with care and with attention to the appropriate modifications.

Glossary

Advanced Program: a demanding program of exercises that shows Pilates as it was intended to be: dynamic, strong and challenging. The advanced exercises should be added to your Intermediate program in order, one by one, when your body is ready to face the challenge.

Ballistic: used to describe movement that is generated using momentum and increasing speed rather than control and precision.

bearing down: forcibly pressing the spine on to a mat with the abdominal muscles bulging, usually while holding the breath in. This will put pressure on the pelvic floor, does not engage the correct muscles and will not be sustainable when you breathe out.

Beginner's Program: the introductory program of Pilates that teaches you how to begin to use the powerhouse to stabilize the lower back and pelvis during movement, and also prepares you for more demanding moves later on. The Pilates principles, particularly control and centering, are introduced with these excercises.

Cautions: points to be aware of in each exercise if you have a particular weakness, limitation or health issue.

C-curve: the position the spine adopts in certain moves so it resembles a capital letter C. The powerhouse lifts the spine so each vertebra is separated and the ribs are lifted off the pelvis, with the abdominals pulled deeply into the spine.

Centering: one of the six Pilates principles referring to working from your center (your powerhouse and centerline) and is associated with being mentally focused and in the moment as you practice Pilates.

Centerline: the midline of the body, from the top of the head, through the nose, breast bone, tummy button, pubic bone and equal distance between the ankles.

Common errors: errors that frequently occur when the Pilates exercises are performed. Being aware of these will help to avoid moving incorrectly and will enable you to move with more precision.

Contrology: the original name for what is today known as Pilates.

core stability: describes the deep abdominal, back and pelvic floor muscles that are active and work in coordination with one another and with more superficial muscles to provide a strong core for a strong body.

'effort with ease': movements that are smooth and flowing and that avoid clenching, bracing, straining and breath-holding.

Elders: some of the original students of Joseph Pilates, who were chosen by him to pass on his methods, beliefs and principles.

endorphins: naturally occurring chemicals released by the brain during exercise that aid pain relief and produce feelings of well-being.

flex: to bend a joint, usually in toward the body. In the ankle the foot lifts up toward the lower leg.

Fundamentals: preliminary Pilates exercises that teach you how to align yourself on the mat and how to scoop your abdominal muscles to stabilize your back and pelvis, while gently imposing movement on top. They educate correct movement patterns to override faulty movement patterns and will aid in learning the bigger movements.

gluteal muscles: three large muscles that make up the buttocks that have two important roles; they move the leg out to the back and the side but also stabilize the pelvis when standing and walking.

hip flexors: strong dominant muscles in the trunk and the thigh that bend the hip, bringing the leg closer to the body. They can become tight through prolonged sitting and poor posture.

holistic: treating the whole person—mind, body and spirit—instead of treating just one system of the body singularly without being aware of the impact the specific condition may have on the other systems of the body. Treating an individual holistically considers how they function as a whole.

iliotibial band: a thick fibrous band that runs from the pelvis to the knee. Large muscles around the hip and pelvis attach to the iliotibial band and it is involved in movement and stability at the hip and the knee.

imprinting: holding the spine softly against the mat, when lying down, so that it does not arch off the mat or bear down with bulging abdominals, forcing the back into the mat.

Intermediate Program: a series of more demanding exercises than those in the Beginner's Program, which challenges you to start moving with flow, greater precision and concentration, getting your breath working with the exercise.

mind–body–spirit modality: a holistic method that encompasses all three aspects of health, rather than isolated or disconnected conditions.

mindfulness: the state of being present in the here and now, to the exclusion of other distractions.

Modifications: variations on the exercises, which you can follow in order to adapt them to your own requirements; use them to enable you to perform an exercise safely or as building blocks to help you, in time, achieve the ideal form of the exercise.

neutral pelvis: when the pelvis is in a midway position—neither tucked under or rolled forward.

neutral spine: the position the spine adopts with natural body curves; when lying on the mat gravity will soften the natural curves and the hollow in the low back will be less, but will be neither arched or forced down onto the mat.

osteopenia: a condition in which bone density is lower than normal, it can often be seen as a precursor to osteoporosis (see below).

osteoporosis: a condition in which the bones have become less dense due to loss of bone minerals, leading to an increased risk of fracture.

oxygenation: the process by which oxygen is absorbed into different parts of the body.

pelvis: three different bones joined together to form a ring and connects the trunk to the legs, the spine connects to the pelvis via the sacrum and the femurs form the hip joint with the pelvis.

Pilates stance: the position the legs adopt when the back of the thighs and the back-side are active forming a "wrap" (see below), the legs will have a soft turn out with the heels and legs pressed together and the toes gently turned out. Pilates stance can be used when standing upright and when the legs are in the air.

powerhouse: a band around your middle that pertains to the deep abdominal and back muscles, pelvic floor and diaphragm with the other abdominal and back muscles layered on top and is supported by the buttocks and inner thighs.

Precision points: pointers to be able to achieve accuracy for each exercise; these will help you to work toward the ideal form of each exercise.

progression signs: indicators that you are strong enough to move from one Pilates level to the next.

proprioception: awareness of where the parts of your body are, and where the whole of your body is in space, helping you to gain balance in your body and control of movement.

quadriceps: a group of four muscles at the front of the thigh.

sacrum: a solid triangular bone located at the base of the spine and connects to the pelvis by the sacro-iliac joint.

scoliosis: a condition in which there is side-to-side curvature of the spine.

scooping: the action of pulling the abdominals inward and upward to help stabilize the spine and decompress it during movement; it is an aid to good posture.

self-resistance: using one muscle against another; if you work with self-resistance you move strongly resisting your own movement, rather than moving loosely, freely, with uncontrolled limbs.

sitting bones: two bones of the pelvis that you are aware of in your buttocks when sitting, balancing and rocking.

tailbone: the small triangular bone, properly known as the coccyx, at the base of the spine.

Transition: a movement that enables you to flow smoothly from one exercise to the next; it encourages you to keep your powerhouse engaged throughout the entirety of a workout.

Visualization: imagery as an aid to learning the correct manner in which to move when doing an exercise; for instance, "Your lungs fill up like two balloons."

wrap: when the back of the thighs and buttocks are engaged which opens the front of the hips and provides a slight turn out of the legs; the wrap helps to support the powerhouse.

zipping up: pulling up between the legs along a strong centerline from the heel to the seat, which pulls up the pelvic floor.

Index

Acknowledgments

Learning Pilates for me has been truly life changing; a real mind, body, spirit experience. Emotional strength has grown with physical confidence and led me to achieve things I didn't know I could. I have met some inspirational people who have believed in me and presented me with opportunities; I am very grateful to these individuals. The energy and drive of my first teacher Lesley McPherson, Gaile Dean who continues to teach and challenge me, to the international trainers who bring Pilates to teachers as a direct lineage from Joseph Pilates, the friends I have made along the journey, particularly Madeleine Brzseki who has always seen more potential in me than I see in myself.

It is also important to acknowledge my physiotherapy colleagues, particularly Miria Putkonen, who have taught, guided and motivated me as the Pilates and physiotherapy have become inseparable in many ways.

Inspiration and motivation also comes from the people whose bodies I treat and teach. In them I see the power that movement can have to heal and increase well-being. Thank you to all my students and patients, I constantly learn from you as I treat or teach you.

My family need to be thanked for their enduring love and patience, most importantly my children Madeline, Isaac and Joseph who are amazing.

A special thank you to Gerry Thompson and to all at Octopus for your guidance and help through this process.

Jo Ferris, who has a graduate diploma in physiotherapy, is a Pilates instructor and physical therapist specializing in neurology at St. Richard's Hospital in Chichester, England. A member of the Chartered Society of Physiotherapists, Ferris teaches Pilates to those who are fit and those who are recovering from injuries.

E-mail: jopilates@virginmedia.com | www.joferris.co.uk

Picture credits: 21 Getty Images/Michael Rougier/Time & Life Pictures; 389 Thinkstock/George Doyle; 391 Corbis/Joan Glase.